Play Helps

To Jill –
So many thanks for all
your inspiration which
has made this possible –
    with love
        from
        Roma.
            Jan 1977

PLAY HELPS
Toys and Activities for Handicapped Children

ROMA LEAR

Illustrated by Gillian Hunter

HEINEMANN HEALTH BOOKS
London

'Heinnemann Health Books' are published
by William Heinemann Medical Books Ltd
23 Bedford Square   London WC1B 3HT

First published 1977

© Roma Lear 1977

ISBN 0 433 19085 X

Typeset by Malvern Typesetting Services
and printed and bound in Great Britain by
Redwood Burn, Trowbridge and Esher

Contents

Foreword

Long before I knew Roma Lear, I knew her letters—the kind you cannot wait to read the moment you recognize the handwriting. Every one of these tightly packed, enthusiastic communications was bursting with suggestions, ideas and reports of the successes and frustrations she was encountering in setting up her Toy Library in Kingston—only the second to open in this country. And there *were* frustrations, disappointments and delays, but these only made its eventual splendid success a greater tribute to Roma's staying powers. This same invaluable capacity for sticking it out and the quiet confidence she conveys to parents too—show the faith, adaptability and resourcefulness we so badly need when faced with our problem handicapped children, with no guarantee from doctors of their eventual potential, and no one offspring ever quite like another. Moreover, her long experience of a wide range of handicaps enables her always to give exceptionally knowledgeable advice. Added to this she is one of those creative people who are at the same time so practical that their ideas never fail to work, and can be copied in the knowledge that every possible snag has been anticipated and forestalled!

Roma and I finally met by accident in Galt's toy shop. She was busily sifting out with wary selectiveness the items her then small toy library budget would run to for the greatest benefit to each of her young clientele—because it is never a case of 'what he *ought* to enjoy' with Roma, but of discovering at first hand what each child will really respond to, however illogical this may sometimes be! She represents superbly one of our first objectives in forming toy libraries—an opportunity for more informal professional support for parents outside either classroom or clinic. More recently, she has begun to pioneer yet another possibility—putting into practice the idea that each toy library could become a local centre for the handicapped on

FOREWORD

which all kinds of community support can focus. She is organizing a community project in Kingston whereby pensioners, school children, youth organizations and interested individuals can make play material for handicapped and sick children, demonstrating to other toy libraries how this can be used to benefit those at the giving as well as at the receiving end.

Alongside these many activities Roma is a home tutor to handicapped children, a keen viola player and a busy mother of a young family. We can count it our great good fortune that she has still found the time and perseverence to share her ideas in a book which is vivid in its anecdotes of children and what can be done for them once we have insight into their needs. This insight she gives us with humour, enabling us to observe much more carefully for ourselves in the future. It is because these needs are paradoxically *not* always apparent, even to those devoted to the children, that so many people will benefit from this book. Not just parents, but child minders of all ages, play group and opportunity class leaders, young teachers, hospital volunteers, health visitors and, one hopes as much as anyone, the nurses and child care officers who have responsibility for handicapped or sick children in full residential care—whether in hospitals, hostels, homes or special schools—where there is such a tremendous need to make enriching and enjoyable every 'lonely uneventful day and long weekend' so well described in 'The Empty Hours' by Maureen Oswin, (Pelican Books 1973). Looking ahead to the days when toy libraries have hobby and play 'clubs' attached to them (because, after all, the toys are only a first stepping stone to other forms of play,) this book will surely become a treasured handbook for every toy library organizer too.

When Heinemann first approached me about producing a book on choosing toys and activities for handicapped children, I knew that no one could produce one so worthwhile as Roma, and as a parent I also knew how important it was that something should be written, and that we did not lose the opportunity Heinemann had given us. Therefore, no one could be more grateful to Roma Lear than I, for having been prepared to undertake the task in her highly practical and knowledgeable way. Her book will compel everyone who reads it, I am sure, to put extra effort into planning the play of both mildly and severely handicapped children alike.

Jill Norris

Introduction

Since I finished my teacher training in 1944 I have been particularly interested in play for handicapped children. As a hospital teacher most of my time was taken up with school activities, but sometimes these had to go by the board. Most of the children in the ward might be of pre-school age, or perhaps in pain or discomfort and therefore much more in need of distraction than 'learning'. I began increasingly to realize that my job did not finish at three-thirty when the tea was wheeled in. From then until bed-time and before school the next day were long hours when some of the children would be intolerably bored and probably very naughty! Those over the acute stage of their illness or accident were desperate for something interesting to do, and I found myself devising activities which they could manage on their own or with a ward friend.

After sixteen years of teaching in various hospitals all ages of children, (some lying in difficult positions, perhaps with legs on traction, one arm out of use, or unable to turn their heads,) I learnt, by using tapes, clothes pegs, magnets and safety pins, to invent ways of keeping pencils to hand and all else from falling off the bed.

Then I 'retired' to have our family and like many Mums with young children, became involved with a playgroup. At first this was in a neighbour's house for a few children who lived in the road, and then we graduated to a much larger one for a group of boisterous under fives. Many of the more energetic ideas in this book date from about this time so parents of lively pre-school children may well find some new ways of amusing them.

When our youngest had started at her first school I chanced to switch on the radio and heard Mrs Jill Norris speak about the Toy Library for handicapped children she had recently started at Enfield. We began a stimulating correspondence and soon I found I had begun a Toy Library at Kingston! Since those early days Toy Libraries have gone

INTRODUCTION

from strength to strength and are now spreading rapidly throughout the British Isles and overseas. At our Toy Library, listening to parents telling me about their children, I realize just how difficult it can sometimes be to find the right toy to be a 'winner'. Perhaps the child is too large—or the toy too small! That can usually be put right by finding (or making) a jumbo version. Perhaps the toy is too delicate, too heavy or too bulky, or perhaps the child only likes cars and refuses to take an interest in anything else. Perhaps, quite simply, he just refuses to take an interest! Every time the Toy Library is open I seem to have a scribble in my notebook to remind me to try to do something about someone's problem. Parents who do not have access to a Toy Library may not know of the many splendid toys on the market. Amongst all the information at the back of this book is a list of toy manufacturers and suppliers who will send toys by post. The Toy Libraries Association publishes an up to date ABC of specially recommended toys which have been found to be particularly successful and popular with handicapped children. They also publish leaflets for parents who want help with play for a child with a particular disability such as deafness, blindness, poor hand function, etc., and a letter of enquiry plus a stamped addressed envelope to The Director, Toy Libraries Association, Sunley House, Gunthorpe Street, London, E1 7RW will bring an up to date price list of publications, and information about the nearest Toy Library.

Many people believe that handicapped children should play with 'normal' toys. In theory I share this view, but in practice I sometimes find it must be a goal to work towards. We all know every child is different (which is a very good thing!) but if you compare a class of five year olds in a First School with the same age group in a Special School you will see at once that for some of them their play needs may well be quite different. There is no point in discussing all these differences. Every parent and Toy Library organizer can think of their own particular 'challenge' and probably no two will be exactly alike. In this book you will find a collection of toys (nearly all home-made) and activities (most of which use 'natural objects' or things found around most homes) all of which have *worked for some children*.

One of my biggest problems has been trying to fit all the ideas into some sort of logical order. After many unsuccessful attempts someone suggested I wrote them on cards and shuffled them about until they began to classify themselves. This seemed to be the answer. It occurred to me that the book could be arranged rather like a recipe book, but instead of soups, fish, meat, etc., play ideas could be

INTRODUCTION

assembled under the names of the five senses. After all, being handicapped implies that one or more of these may not be as efficient as it should be, therefore any attractive activity that helps a child to improve his use of that sense must surely be to his advantage. I hope that by this classification parents can quickly dip into the book and find an idea which could be just right for their particular child. For example, a child with poor vision may not enjoy the looking games, but could have plenty of fun feeling and listening, a young profoundly deaf child may miss out on parts of the chapter on hearing while parents of physically handicapped children and slow learners may find some new ideas in all the chapters. There are also suggestions for games and activities which all the family can share, irrespective of age or handicap. Each chapter has been arranged approximately in chronological order, so parents of babies and young children will find the early parts of each the most useful.

This book has been written primarily for parents, who, after all, usually spend more time with their child than anyone else. Many Mums and Dads have the added challenge of having to provide stimulating opportunities for play for both handicapped and 'normal' children, and I hope they will rootle through the pages and find some new ideas that will lead to many happy playtimes.

I have tried to include only those ideas which can work satisfactorily without too much fuss and expense. I am sure many readers will have their own pet play standbys, and I would be delighted to hear about these and pass them on to other parents.

My grateful thanks to all those children over the years who have unwittingly supplied the material for this book, to my family for all their help and forbearance, to Jill Norris and my many friends in the Toy Libraries Association, particularly Susan Knowles and Jean Hemens for their advice on play for deaf and blind children, to Mrs Olwen Marston of Freshwater (Isle of Wight) Women's Institute for her pattern of the Chatty Chick which has brought pleasure to so many children, and to Gillian Hunter for her delightful illustrations.

ROMA LEAR

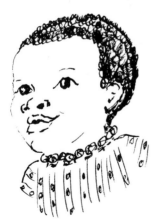

1 Making the most of SIGHT

Although this chapter is written for all children with any degree of vision, however slight, it is intended to be particularly helpful for parents and others concerned with the care of severely physically handicapped, delicate, sick, slow-learning and deaf children.

THE IMPORTANCE OF LEARNING TO LOOK

Any handicapped child needs to be given many opportunities for just *looking.* For those children who find it difficult to concentrate or take an interest in their environment a special effort is needed to provide them with things they will really want to look at. For all children situations ought to be created for them to build up their own store of visual impressions. This might well be by arranging visits to interesting places. A child who has been taken to the zoo and had fun feeding buns to the elephants will have a much better idea of the size and shape of these particular animals than if he had merely seen them in two dimensions in a picture book. The living creature makes much more compelling viewing than the image on the flat page.

As well as providing worthwhile looking it is also very important to provide the time to enjoy it all. The well-known poem 'Leisure' by W. H. Davies tells of many pleasures that are there for those who have eyes to see them, but when we are grown up, caring for a family and home, opportunities (and often the desire) to 'stand and stare' may no longer be there. We constantly tell our children to 'come along' and 'hurry up'. The temptation to chivvy is all the stronger in a large family where the pace must frequently be regulated to that of the slowest member. Adults make time to look when they visit art galleries and exhibitions and are enriched by what they see. Children rely on *us* to provide them with such opportunities.

Apart from the obvious pleasure we all get from looking at beautiful and interesting things, it is vital for purely practical reasons to help a handicapped child to make the best possible use of his eyes. Imagine the problems of a deaf child. He must be encouraged to be extra observant to make up for his defective ears. He cannot hear the lorry coming; he must be trained to look. He cannot hear us when we call him so he must learn to watch, and see when we want to communicate. Slow-learners too need much encouragement to use their eyes so that they can really make use of what they see. Some children may only stare and seldom really *look.* The information their eyes can give makes very little impression on them. Others are so busy looking they seldom *see* but flutter like a butterfly from one object to another without really noticing anything. Perhaps such a child from either of these groups is playing on the grass and picks a bunch of daisies. He might enjoy gathering them, but then just throws them down. That could be the end of that, but if he carries the daisies home, arranges them in an egg cup and puts them in the centre of the table for all the family to enjoy he will have been given the opportunity to have at least three good looks at them — when they were picked and selected from among other flowers or blades of grass, when he arranged them (and incidentally found out quite a lot about the different lengths of stems, especially if they did not fit conveniently into the egg cup), and when he put them in the place of honour for everyone to admire. This concentrated looking coupled with the praise and limelight received for his 'flower arrangement' could help him to remember a great deal about the daisy. The three opportunities for such directed observation will have increased his general experience and may well encourage him to further effort another day.

Many a child has natural curiosity, a delight in the ridiculous, and intense concentration when his attention has really been captured. When he is shown a pretty little ornament, something precious or old, has been taken to visit an interesting place, or simply has his attention drawn to a spectacular sunset he may be building up associations and memories which might influence his life more than we can perhaps imagine. Everyone is likely to have periods of time when he must be alone. Then those with lively minds and a good store of experiences and memories are at a great advantage.

Many years ago Rachel, a frail, shy little girl, lay on her plaster shell in the middle of a noisy orthopædic ward. Certainly she was never alone but because she was artistic and thoughtful perhaps she was one of the loneliest children there. She had spent nearly all of her eleven years in hospital, only going home occasionally for short visits. One afternoon she was given a brand new packet of Plasticene with all the colours still in their corrugated strips, a tray to work on, some white paper, scissors, crayons and some cocktail sticks. By the end of the afternoon she had made an exquisite model of the seaside complete with ice cream van, bathing tents and boats. There was Dad lying on the sand with his trouser legs rolled up and the newspaper over his face. Mum sat beside him surrounded by mounds of clothing and picnic bric-à-brac. Children paddled and dug and tunnelled in the sand. A dog was running off with a ball and a fat little baby was crawling towards the sea with big sister running after him. The whole scene was so alive and full of humour that I have remembered it for thirty years. Rachel told me she had spent a day at Brighton. Her hungry little mind had soaked up like a sponge all the things she saw and she was able to re-create that special day for her own delight — and mine.

LEARNING TO LOOK

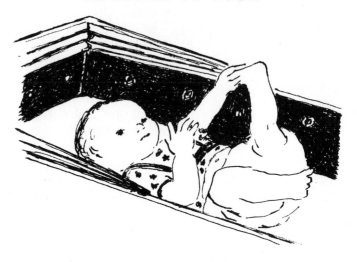

Imagine you are watching a contented little baby lying quietly in his pram, under a tree in the garden. The sun makes flecked shadows across the side of the pram and the baby pats the plastic lining as he tries to catch them. The shadows mottle the back of his hand and he turns his fist this way and that, trying to puzzle out why his skin looks different in shade or in sunlight. His mother begins to hang up the washing. He spends a long time watching her, fascinated by the shapes and colours she is pegging up. He waves his hands and feet and stops to capture and suck a chubby big toe. A breeze makes the thinner pieces of washing flap a little, like a giant mobile. The gentle noise and movement attracts his attention. Looking up at the washing line helps our baby to notice the clouds. Today they are like soft little blobs of cotton wool, and he is fascinated by the way they seem to disappear over the roof of the house. A bird flies across the garden. It is too quick for baby to follow but now it sits singing on the branch of a tree. He turns his head and sees the bird before it flies on to the next branch. The breeze catches a bunch of ribbons tied to the side of the pram hood and he tries to catch them. He sees the studs holding the lining of his pram in place and rolls on his side in order to reach them. He pokes them with a fat little finger trying to score a bull's eye every time. He perseveres until he has several successes. He yawns.

Heigh-ho, it's been a busy morning. Time for a nap!

This baby has had plenty to watch and to interest him. Soon he will be sitting up, crawling, walking and climbing. With each of these activities he will find fresh things to look at. For handicapped children this may not be so. Their time for sitting, crawling and walking may be delayed by months, even years. Some will never move independently. Others may have limited movement with snags attached. The young spina bifida child on his little trolley can change his position within a room, giving himself a splendid view of knees and table legs, but he cannot see out of the window to watch life in the street or admire his big brother making a model on the dining-room table. The child in a wheel-chair, even if he can propel it himself, is limited to flat surfaces and slopes. Other children need to lie in a particular position or even to see the world in reverse with the help of a mirror. Whatever the problem, something worthwhile for them to watch must surely be found.

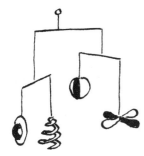

THINGS FOR AN IMMOBILE CHILD TO WATCH

Suspended Toys

Just hanging up a favourite doll or teddy by a length of elastic can often help a child to see it in a different way. To make more compulsive viewing it can be made to bounce, or pushed to make it revolve gently.

A Bunch of Balloons

Balloons are cheap, large and colourful and seem to appeal to all children. They will stir with the slightest draught and this movement will help to attract a baby's attention. A suspended balloon, not too heavily inflated so that there is little risk of it popping, can have a few grains of rice or even a small budgerigar bell inside. This turns it into a kind of giant rattle and children with poor co-ordination often enjoy trying to hit it. The rewarding noise adds to the fun.

Bubbles

Blown across a cot by an adult or older child, these have delighted many a baby. Care must be taken to avoid the bubbles popping in his face. Washing up liquid, slightly diluted, makes an excellent bubble mixture and a few drops of glycerine or cooking oil added to it help to make the bubbles stronger. A wand to dip in the mixture and shake can be made from a piece of wire or a pipe cleaner. Bend one end into a circle to make a shape like a lollipop. Dip the loop in the mixture and wave it about or blow gently through it to make the bubbles. Alternatively a cotton reel can be dipped in the liquid and a bubble blown through the hole. Some small children love to blow bubbles this way. If they blow towards the floor they will avoid getting a mouthful of detergent which can easily happen if they try to use a bubble pipe and suck by mistake!

Mobiles

These are popular with children of all ages and many older ones and parents enjoy creating their own. Suggestions and hints on making mobiles can be found on page 47. Attractive readymade ones can be bought at many toy and baby shops or through the toy suppliers listed on page 153.

GAMES WHICH ENCOURAGE CHILDREN TO LOOK

Peep Bo

This old favourite has been enjoyed by babies from time immemorial. It is the element of anticipation and surprise which they find so delightful, and a resourceful parent can make use of this appeal. A teddy who pops up from behind the back of an armchair, sometimes over the top, sometimes round the side, will often hold a child's attention for a surprisingly long time.

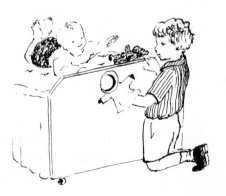

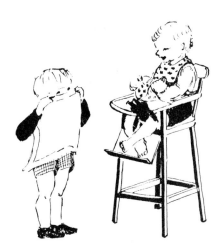

The King of the Castle Lost His Hat

Everyone knows the time-honoured game of 'I Spy with my little Eye' where one player says the initial letter of an object and the other players must try to guess what he has spied. This game is excellent for encouraging a child to look around and notice things, but it is too difficult for young children, or for older ones who have not learnt about letter sounds. 'The King of the Castle Lost His Hat' only requires a child to be able to recognize some colours, and the game can be made as simple as is necessary. The leader thinks of an object in the room. It could be the carpet, or a cushion, or a ribbon in someone's hair. He then says the nonsense rhyme—

The King of the Castle lost his hat,

Some say this and some say that,

But I say Mr Green (or Blue, or Red, etc. according to the colour of the object he has chosen). The other children must try to guess the 'green' thing. The person who gets it right takes over as leader for the next turn. As skill increases the colours can be made more difficult, e.g. Mr Black and Silver might be the knob on the television set.

Searching Games

All searching games like 'Hunt the Thimble' or 'Hide and Seek' are good for encouraging children to look more carefully. A popular game to while away a long car journey can be looking out of the window for certain landmarks or easily spotted objects like a letter box or a blue car. This game can be useful on walks too. Town

7

children can watch a busy road for interesting vehicles and country children can look for natural objects. Some children enjoy a treasure hunt where they can be asked to find particular things like a round stone, or a yellow flower, or something square.

Christmas Card Jig-saws The simplest game is to cut two cards in half, one straight down the middle and the other diagonally across. Let the child match the halves to remake the pictures.

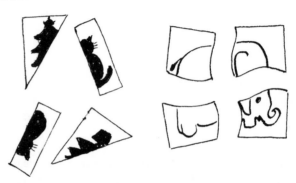

A more complicated puzzle can be made by cutting one card into several pieces which the child must fit together again. The task is even more challenging if two cards are cut up and the pieces muddled together for the child to sort out.

To make this kind of puzzle easier to handle and more robust glue the front and the back of the card together before you cut it into shapes.

Kim's Game This is a game requiring keen observation and a good memory, but it can easily be adapted to meet the needs of children of varying ages or degrees of intelligence. It is usually played as a group game, but works just as well with one child and an adult.

The basic game Arrange some easily recognized objects on a tray, e.g. a match box, cotton reel, thimble, small toy, button, pencil, etc. The number of objects chosen will depend on the ability of the child. He then has a little while to take a look at all the objects and memorize their position on the tray. He hides his eyes while one object is removed. When he opens them he has another look at the tray and guesses which object is missing.

Variations

Instead of taking something off the tray another object can be added, or the position of two objects can be changed. The child must then guess which ones have been moved.

Sometimes a child can help to collect the objects for the tray, perhaps choosing all round shaped things, or rectangular ones, or those of a particular colour. Because he has contributed to the selection, a child with a poor memory will have a better chance of identifying the items in the game.

Simple Ball Games

Ball games are often a child's first experience of playing an organized game with someone else. While the play lasts, child and adult have each other's undivided attention and both can find this very enjoyable.

Rolling Games

All ball games are excellent for encouraging children to look, and it is not hard to adapt ball play to the requirements of almost any child. At first, slowly rolling a ball across the floor, aiming for a baby's hand, will give him the idea of the game. He may want to chew and fondle the ball at first, but he will gradually learn to try to return it when he realizes it will be bowled to him again. Providing there is no physical reason why he should not adopt this position, sitting the child with his legs apart can make a sort of harbour for the ball, and gives him a better chance to grab it. If he will only use one hand, and it is desirable to encourage him to use both, the ball can be aimed at the 'good' hand until he learns to watch for it coming, and then aimed occasionally at the 'lazy' hand to persuade him to use that too.

A large ball, such as an inflatable beach ball, can also be helpful, for the size of the ball makes him need two hands to control it.

Playing Goal Keeper

This is another good way of helping a child to watch a moving ball. He stands in a doorway, supporting himself by the doorposts if he finds it difficult to balance while he kicks, and the ball can be rolled towards him along the hall or landing (as long a distance as possible so that he has plenty of time to watch it coming).

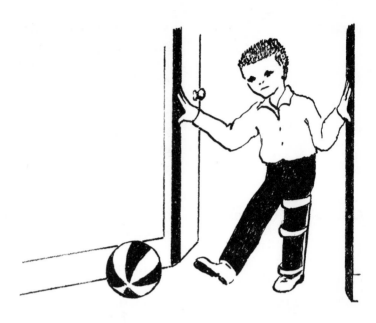

Throwing and Catching Games

When rolling games have become boring it is time to move on to the more difficult skills of throwing and catching. Sometimes it is easier for a child to manage a bean bag or a small cushion which does not roll away. Brightly coloured inflatable plastic beach balls are large and light and the most suitable for some children; others may find the Airfix plastic foam ball easier to manage. It is about the size of a large grapefruit, and because it is squashy it can be grasped firmly and does not spring out of the fingers. An 'instant' ball can be made by rolling up a pair of socks, or by stuffing the toe of a stocking with crunched up pieces of newspaper. The stocking is twisted round just above the newspaper and turned inside out so that it covers the stuffed toe again. Repeat the twisting and recovering until the stocking is used up and the ball is covered with many layers. A few quick stitches or dabs of fabric adhesive will secure the top.

Toss in the Bin

The ball must be thrown into a grocery carton or a waste paper basket with the child standing close at first, and gradually moving further away as he becomes more skillful. A generous supply of balls is required and those made from newspaper and old stockings (described above) are quite suitable.

Aunt Sally

This game is popular at our Toy Library parties which include children of all ages and abilities. A large grocery carton has a cheerful face painted on one side. The mouth is cut away to make a large hole through which bean bags can be thrown. A bell is suspended from the roof of the box like a giant epiglottis and every time a bean bag sails through the mouth the bell rings, signalling success!

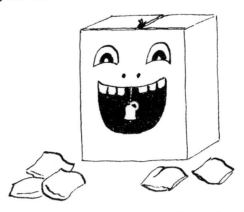

Throwing Ping Pong Balls into Jam Jars

This is a popular money raiser at fêtes, but it is also a game that can be enjoyed at home. The ping pong balls jump out of the jars unless very carefully aimed, and the game calls for considerable skill and luck. The jars can be numbered and scores kept. Yogurt pots make good substitutes for jam jars and avoid using glass which can be dangerous. Should the yogurt pots topple over too easily they can be weighed down with a few pebbles in the bottom. If ping pong balls are not handy large buttons, butter beans, etc can be thrown instead.

Clock Golf

Once a child has learnt to aim, more organized games become possible. These can often be a good way of helping a handicapped child to play on an equal footing with other children. A useful game to start with can be Clock Golf. This needs an area of fairly smooth grass, and the correct equipment for marking out the game can be bought at sports shops, but for children making their first attempts to play it an improvised course will do just as well. Before beginning the game the pitch must be marked out like a clock face, with the numbers one to twelve evenly spaced around the circumference of a

11

circle. In the centre where the hands would be fixed, a small hole must be sunk. The players take it in turns to stand on each number (starting with one,) and must hit a ball into the central hole using as few strokes as possible. This game is also most suitable for playing on a sandy beach where a bucket can be sunk to make the hole, and the numbers can either be drawn in the sand or marked by cairns of stones. The real game is played with golf balls and putters, but children can be quite content to use walking sticks and tennis balls.

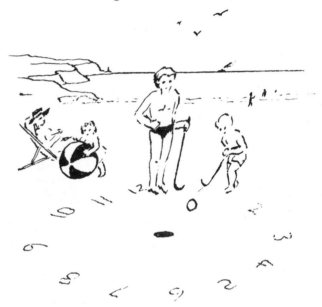

HELPING OLDER CHILDREN TO MAKE THE MOST OF SIGHT

Television must surely top the popularity poll as a looking activity, but even this can pall at times and suitable programmes are not always available. At its best television is stimulating and extending as well as being entertaining. At its worst it can merely kill time, and children have been known to spend minutes just staring at the test card! The following suggestions may help to offer an attractive alternative.

A Looking Corner

In many a Nursery School, Playgroup and First School you will find a table set aside for things that are chosen specially to be looked at. This is an idea well worth imitating at home. Perhaps part of a shelf or a window ledge might be a suitable place to display a few interesting exhibits. These must be changed as soon as they no longer attract attention. Objects to put in a looking corner might include a model made by the child and one or two very special things. These might perhaps be fragile, or unusual, or ring the changes between a collection of shells, leaves, flowers, photographs, red things, blue things, heavy or light things, floating or flying things . . . the list of possibilities is very long and elastic.

Going on a Seeing Saunter

So often a walk is a matter of necessity—perhaps going to meet a child from school or to do the shopping, but sometimes it is an excellent idea to take a long time going nowhere in particular. On such walks town children can discover different designs on the brickwork of houses, patterns on drain covers, numbers on gates, plants growing in peculiar places etc, and there are many interesting things to see on a busy road. Country children can look for flowers, leaves or pretty stones, or can search for insects. They will find plenty of treasures once they have learnt to look properly.

Pets

Because of their unpredictability and constant movement, animals, birds and fish are always fascinating to watch, and they can make ideal companions for many handicapped children. The following outline of the kind of care certain creatures need is intended for parents who have not yet kept a pet but are considering adding one to the family. Much fuller information can be had from pet shops which sell paperbacks about all pets, and of course from public libraries and pet clubs.

Goldfish

These are the easiest to care for and only need a large plastic tank, some special grit for the bottom and a carton of fish food which lasts for a very long time. Once happily installed fish need very little care. The water must be kept pure and slime cleaned from the

13

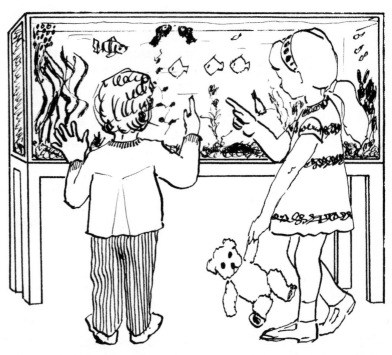

sides of the tank when necessary. The fish like a little food daily and appreciate some water weeds to swim through, but should they *occasionally* be forgotten they will survive quite well. They have been known to live for fifteen years or more.

Caged birds

Popular in many hospital wards these have certain advantages as pets. They are colourful and attractive to listen to, and have more personality than fish. They require daily care which includes feeding, watering and cleaning out, but all of this can be accomplished by many handicapped children in a few moments. A bird will possibly live for as long as ten years.

Attracting and watching wild birds

This can be a worthwhile and absorbing hobby. Even in a home that has a cat a safe bird table can often be arranged, either on a pole within clear view of a downstairs window or fixed to an upstairs window ledge or to a balcony rail. Children love to thread peanuts in their shells to make a special 'necklace' for the tits, or to make a bird pudding. Into this can go chopped scraps of meat and fat, dried bread, a few raisins or raw peanuts (not salted ones) odd bits of bacon rind, biscuit crumbs, left overs from the bottom of cereal packets, oatmeal etc. Ideally these should be minced to stop the greedy birds from taking the biggest pieces. The mixture can be put into a basin and melted dripping (which need not be very hot) must be poured over it to stick it all together. Press it down and leave it to set. This wierd concoction can be cut into slices and fed to the birds. It is sure to be popular with a wide variety of species.

Using a mincer can be very dangerous if one child is allowed to turn the handle while another feeds in the food. If one child does both operations, pushing the food onto the mincing screw with a cotton reel or a small wooden spoon, so keeping his fingers well clear, he can regulate the speed with which he turns the handle to suit his own pace. Seeing the food come out in tiny pieces gives children a big thrill, and done under supervision in the way suggested it is reasonably safe.

Birds love a bath and a dish of water on the bird table will attract them almost as much as food. An old tin plate with a stone in it to stop it tipping up will serve very well, but a perfect bird bath can be made from an old metal dustbin lid supported on some bricks. Smaller birds can flutter at the edge while the larger ones will choose to wallow in the middle.

In springtime a bird's nest building rack is a thing many children enjoy making. A strip of onion netting (begged from the greengrocer) can be attached to a piece of wood top and bottom, to straighten it out and weight it down like a wall hanging. Scraps of wool, hay, feathers etc. can be poked into the net fairly firmly, threading them in and out, so that they will not fall off but will be ready for the first bird in search of building material. The net can be hung from a convenient tree. The bottom edge must also be tethered so that the net does not sway too violently in the wind and the birds must be given time to get used to it before they are expected to help themselves to the nesting materials. A necklace of threaded peanuts or any other bird delicacy, like the bone from a joint with a few scraps of meat still on it, hung at the side of the net may help to attract the birds to it.

The Royal Society for the Protection of Birds, The Lodge, Sandy, Bedfordshire SG19 2DL encourages children to be bird watchers. The Society publishes a book called 'The Birds in your Garden' which is of particular interest to children, and a list of more detailed books on ornithology. It can supply bird posters and charts, gramophone records of bird song, models to make and games that help in learning to recognize different species. Garden bird equipment like nesting boxes and bird tables are also quoted on the price list and the Society runs a Young Ornithologists Club.

Animals

These can make wonderful companions for a handicapped child, and the more he can share in the care and attention they need the closer the friendship between them will grow. Some animals obviously require more attention than others, but all need regular feeding, cleaning out and grooming. Parents understand the care they must be prepared to give to a cat or dog, and may feel they cannot spare the time or energy for these pets. They may like to consider other smaller furry animals which are entertaining to watch and lovely to hold once they have been tamed. A garden and a draught-free dry shed for the cage in winter make the keeping of rabbits and guinea pigs a possibility. Gerbels, mice and hamsters (much more restless little creatures which are most lively at night time) need to be kept indoors in the warm, but if they are healthy and cleaned out frequently they should not smell. They need plenty of gentle care and handling if they are to become really tame and companionable. Wire and metal cages are suitable for these small animals. Rabbits and guinea pigs need bigger wooden hutches. These larger animals can cost quite a lot to keep and before deciding to buy one it is as well to enquire at a pet shop for the current prices of seed, hay and straw for bedding, and wood chips or sawdust for the bottom of the cage. They also need crunchy fresh food such as cabbage, lettuce, carrot, apple, celery etc.

Wild pets are kept by most country children at some time or another, and these can be lovely things to watch for a short time. Unfortunately the mortality rate can be very high if, for instance, minnows from a running stream are kept in stagnant water in a jam jar, or caterpillars are incarcerated in a dark, airless shoe box, and it is distressing for children to see the dead creatures they have unwittingly killed. It is much better to catch the fish or insect, HAVE A GOOD LOOK and then let it go again. Snails and caterpillars will live happily for a little while in a shoe box kept in a cool place (not on a sunny window ledge) with a piece of old net curtain tied over the top. Caterpillars can also be kept for a short time on a branch of their natural food. To do this use two jam jars. Fill one with water and cover the top with a piece of cardboard with a hole in the middle. Poke the end of the twig holding the caterpillars through the cardboard into the water. Cover

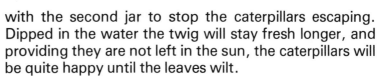

with the second jar to stop the caterpillars escaping. Dipped in the water the twig will stay fresh longer, and providing they are not left in the sun, the caterpillars will be quite happy until the leaves wilt.

Tadpoles seem to make the best 'wild pets' and will hatch out of their cluster of jelly very satisfactorily. They seem to enjoy being kept in a large jar or goldfish bowl in a shady place, and wiggle energetically in and out of a bit of pond weed. They appreciate a pinch of goldfish food occasionally. When their legs have grown it is time to let them go back to their pond.

WATCHING PLANTS GROW

The main disadvantage of growing things is the length of time it takes to see any spectacular result, but older children who have learnt to be more patient can find great pleasure and satisfaction in tending them and watching the gradual development of a tiny seed into a flourishing plant.

Using Vegetables

An *onion* can be rested on the neck of a jam jar filled with water. Place it on a sunny window ledge and keep the water topped up. Soon roots will grow and the onion will sprout leaves. One grown like this has even been known to flower! Other bulbs such as hyacinths can be grown this way but these take longer to sprout than onions. Even an acorn will eventually develop roots and shoots. Balance this, scarred end downwards, on the neck of a bottle filled with water.

Tops of carrots, parsnips, beetroot and turnips can all be made to grow more leaves. The cut surface must be kept in a saucer of water and never allowed to dry out. Growth is fairly rapid and the first signs of new leaves can be expected after a very few days.

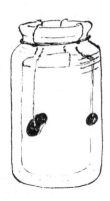

Peas and beans can be grown in a jam jar with a cylinder of damp blotting paper in the middle to keep them moist. The dried peas and beans should be soaked over night to help them to germinate more quickly. When they are just poked round the sides of the jar between the glass and the blotting paper they tend to fall to the bottom and it is not easy to see the way the roots and leaves grow from the seeds. It is worth the extra effort to thread each seed on a length of cotton. Dangle them until they hang about half way down inside the jar and fix the thread to the outside with sticky tape until they are arranged satisfactorily (e.g. two peas and two beans opposite each other.) Wind some wool firmly round the neck of the jar to hold the threads securely, put the roll of blotting paper inside the jar and make sure it is always kept damp. After a few days the seeds will start to sprout and children love to watch to see which will grow the fastest.

Fruit pips can be planted in a little soil, which is damp but not soggy. Enclosed in a polythene bag and kept on a sunny window sill, the seed will germinate in time. Orange pips look very pretty growing in a scooped out half of orange.

See also Cress Hedgehog in 'Taste'. Page 123.

Making a Garden in a Meat Tin

Children enjoy creating their own little gardens, and these can be very decorative when they are finished. Half fill an old meat tin, or any suitable container, with damp earth. Grass can be grown from real seed, or moss can be laid for lawns; a hand bag mirror or a shiny tin lid makes a good pond; twigs from bushes and shrubs can make trees; flowers can be poked into the damp earth, or made to last longer if they are arranged in water in paste jars or thimbles embedded in the soil, and paths

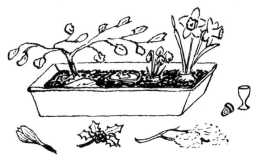

can be made from small stones. A garden such as this would be ideal to grace a looking table (page 13).

Less elaborate gardens can be made in a saucer filled with damp moss or sand. Flowers with fairly thick stems can be poked in and will last well for several hours. Florists sell a green plastic foam substance called Oasis, which is useful for children who particularly enjoy working with flowers.

OTHER ACTIVITIES WHICH ENCOURAGE LOOKING

Playing with Paint

Dabbling with colour seems to have a universal appeal for all sighted children, but sometimes the practical difficulties of providing painting for those at home are so great that many children can miss out on this delightful activity. If you would like to introduce your child to painting but have not yet done so because of the problems you must solve, or if you already have paints in the house but your child is bored with them and you have run out of ideas on how to use them a different way, read on!

PLAY HELPS

Hints for Parents About to Introduce Paint

(1) Choose the right moment. Allow for quite a long session to include time for preparation and clearing up, and if you have a toddler younger than your handicapped child wait until he is in bed or out visiting so that you can concentrate on helping the older one. Before bath time can be a suitable time of the day, and will save you an extra clean up.

(2) Choose the right place—a room with an easily cleaned floor in case of spills, and a large table top so that there is plenty of room to work and paint jars are less likely to be accidentally knocked over.

(3) Check up on your equipment before you start. You will need

a) plenty of protective covering for child, table and floor, and a squeezy cloth at the ready to mop up any spills.

b) suitable paint and brushes. For these first attempts avoid a cheap paint box with hard little cakes of colour. Children lack the patience to stroke the paint onto the brush and the results are often disappointingly pale and watery. Use powder paint which can be bought in small tins at art shops, large stationers or toy shops, and mix it with a little Polycell, Gloy, or homemade flour and water paste (see Basic Recipes page 147). This will stop the paint from dripping off the end of the brush. Non spill paint pots can usually be bought with the powder paints, or they can be improvised from detergent bottles. To make one, cut off the bottom half of the bottle to hold the paint, then cut off the shaped top just below the shoulder of the bottle. Take off the stopper, turn the top upside down and wedge it firmly into the lower part which will contain the paint. (There should be at least an inch between the lip of the funnel and the bottom of the bottle.) The paint container now looks like the shape of an extinct volcano. The child can poke his brush down the central hole and if he knocks the pot over there is usually time to right it before the paint can escape round the edge of the top. The pot can be weighted with a stone inside it to make it less easily knocked over.

Brushes for first attempts need to be fat and easily held. Special ones with long or short handles can be bought with the paints, but some children prefer a decorator's brush or even a piece of dowelling (perhaps the handle of an old washing up mop) with a piece of foam plastic tied securely to one end.

c) a good supply of large sheets of scrap paper.

(4) Be prepared to spend plenty of time with your child until you are sure he can manage on his own.

If you feel that using paint may have too many pitfalls, try a preliminary run using only plain water and a brush until you feel more confident of your child's ability. Many papers will change colour when they are wetted, and your child may well be fascinated by this. Try 'painting' on newspaper, non-shiny notepaper, blotting paper from a finished pad, or even toilet paper though this tears easily.

For a first session in using paint it can be fun to colour the wrong side of heavily embossed wallpaper. Let your child use a very fat brush (or even the foam plastic 'brush' described above,) and have the paint fairly thick and manageable. As the brush is pulled across the paper the 'bumps' will be coloured while the 'dents' remain white. This is a lovely activity for young or less able children who can all produce delightful results at their first attempts.

When your child progresses to using several colours do not be disappointed if he produces completely unrecognizable splodges at first. He will be experimenting and thoroughly enjoying himself and that is really all that matters at this stage!

Hints for Experienced Parents Used to Painting Sessions

The next time your child wants to paint he may have run out of ideas and look to you to start him off on something new and exciting. It is always useful to have some surprises up your sleeve and the following suggestions may remind you of things you enjoyed doing in your childhood, or you may be introduced to some new ways of using paint for fun. They are all well-tried ideas and could provide a happy diversion on a wet day or when your child is feeling a bit 'off colour'.

PLAY HELPS

**Candle grease
Magic Pictures**

With the end of an old candle draw a simple picture on a fairly large piece of paper. Press hard so that the candle grease really rubs off. Your child can cover the paper with a wash of colour, using a watery paint and a thick brush. He will find that the paint does not stick to the grease marks, and he can discover the magic picture. For children who can read it is fun to write a message with the candle, and even an unpopular one like 'Clear up and then go to bed,' has been known to finish a painting session off happily!

Making a Butterfly

Use a piece of shiny paper and fold it in half. Open it out again. On one side of the crease the child paints half a butterfly, using blobs of bold colours, and making the base of the wing touch the crease. The other half of the paper is folded over onto this and rubbed gently to make the paint stick to it. When the paper is opened out there should be a beautiful butterfly with the same pattern on both his wings.

Making Ghosts

This is done in the same way as the butterfly but the blobs of colour are put onto the crease of the paper. When the sides are pressed together the paint will spread into an unpredictable shape. Personal 'ghosts' can be made by writing a name on the fold in joined up writing with plenty of paint and then closing up the paper and pressing it along the crease to spread out the colour.

Making a Rainbow

Collect together the correct colours. All you really need are red, yellow and blue as these can be made to merge together to make all the colours of the rainbow—red, orange, yellow, green, blue, indigo and violet. Let your child make a sheet of paper wet all over, and then paint hoops of colour, starting with red, letting them blend into each other. It is necessary to work fairly quickly before the paper dries out.

Spatter Prints

These are very messy to do, but are great fun and splendid for encouraging a child to use both hands. Even the least able children can produce results as good as those done by the more capable ones so they are excellent for building confidence.

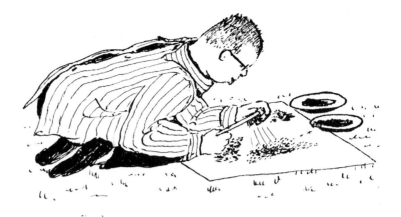

You need plenty of protection for everything—child, walls, floor and table! You also need some paper, an old toothbrush and some paint. The brush is dipped in the paint and held, bristles downwards, fairly close to the paper. As the child runs his fingers along the bristles the paint is spattered (hopefully!) onto it.

Making a Full-length Self Portrait

The child lies on a strip of ceiling paper, or on the back of the remains of a roll of wallpaper. Draw round him with a thick felt pen or a dark crayon. Show him how to colour himself in, and 'hang' him in a place of honour. This activity is excellent for children who have problems with body awareness, and gives them some idea of their size and shape.

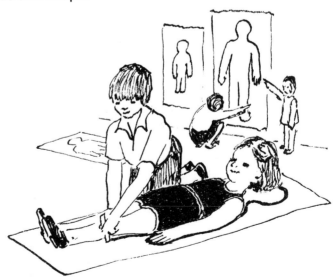

Making Footprints or Gloves for all the Family

This is easier than a full length portrait because only hands or feet are involved. For *footprints* draw round both feet, colour in the outlines and cut them out. Some children like to make plenty of their own footprints on fairly thick paper, cut them out, fasten them to the floor with Blue Tac and walk along them, making their feet fit the prints. This is very good practice in balancing and can help a child to realize the difference between his left and right feet. (Blue Tac is a material rather like Plasticine which can be worked in the fingers until it becomes slightly tacky and soft. It will then stick paper to a smooth surface such as glass, tiles, walls or lino, and will not leave a mark. It can be retrieved at the end of the game and used again another time. It is available from most stationers.)

To make *paper gloves* draw round each hand, colour in the outline and cut out the shape. Young children find it easier to make paper mitts with the fingers joined together and just the thumb drawn round separately. This activity can be turned into a useful sorting game which teaches the word 'pair'. It is of course important that the gloves in each pair should look alike! If left to their own devices, children often do not think of this. Primary colours can be used, or simple striped patterns, or even elaborate 'Fairisle' designs. Incidentally, as a teacher I have used pairs of paper gloves very successfully to explain the building up of the two times table.

Printing

While all kinds of artistic creation using paper and colours will undoubtably encourage a child to look at what he is doing, printing can often have certain extra advantages for handicapped children. If they are prepared to take a little trouble those who are physically incapable of free painting or lack the imagination to make a picture can find great pleasure in printing patterns. Bold results can be produced fairly quickly, but more elaborate prints may need slow, careful sustained effort so that it is an activity that can be made to suit many individual requirements.

Practical Hints

Paper

Avoid glossy paper which tends to reject the paint. Provide as large a piece as is sensible, remembering that some children will be discouraged if they have too big a surface to cover. Newspaper is good for first attempts providing the print is not too obtrusive, but butcher's paper, ceiling lining paper or the back of the remains of a roll of wall paper (without an embossed pattern) are even better. Older children with good hand control enjoy printing on good quality note paper, making small things like Christmas cards, book marks or frames for special photographs.

Paint

For 'messy workers' use a washable powder paint mixed stiffly, and add some wallpaper paste to make it go a little further. Put a pad of cotton wool, or thin foam rubber into an unbreakable dish. An old tin plate, or baking pattypans, or the base of a washing up liquid bottle cut off about 1″ from the bottom would all do very well. The paint container needs to be robust in case an over-enthusiastic child presses too hard. If he uses a china saucer this might be cracked. Pour the paint onto the pad and give it time to soak in. Alternatively, put the pad on a puddle of paint and press down gently until the colour oozes through. The child can now press his printing shape onto the pad and transfer the paint to the paper. Some children prefer to paint the shape every time they use it. They will not need a printing pad but can use poster paint or thick powder paint applied with a brush.

Shapes to Print With

Here the list of possibilities is enormous and children love experimenting with different surfaces and shapes.
Try (a) printing with a part of the body like
—the palm of the hand,
—the tip of a finger or thumb,
—an elbow,
—a foot, heel or toe.
(b) Printing with a soft pad such as
—a ball of cotton wool tied up in a soft rag,
—a foam rubber mopping up cloth tied tightly round a rolled up stocking. (This makes an interesting mottled pattern.)
—a nylon pan scourer which can be wrapped up in rag if the child needs something to take hold of.

(c) Printing with specially prepared shapes, e.g.
—a potato cut in half with a simple shape gouged out from the cut surface,
—a carrot cut in half makes splendid spots,
—an India rubber carved into a clearly defined shape such as a child's initial,
—a string print. For this a short length of string is glued to a block of wood. An old building brick will do. The string must be carefully arranged so that it lies flat and does not cross over itself or the pattern will not print evenly.
—a felt shape, cut from an old hat perhaps, and glued to the end of a cotton reel.

(d) printing with everyday objects.
This is just a question of seeing potential printing shapes in commonplace objects.
To give you some ideas
—the end of a pencil makes small spots;
—the end of a ruler makes short lines;
—the edge of a ruler makes long lines;
—a cotton reel makes a good wheel shape;
—a leaf, the head of a screw, half a clothes peg etc. can all be used to print interesting shapes.

Preparation for Printing

If a paint pad is used the process should not be too messy, but prepare for the worst by protecting the table top and floor with plenty of newspaper. Many parents find that an old plastic raincoat or a shirt worn back to front and tied round the child's waist makes an ideal protector for him.

Using Printing for Fun

Young children are quite happy to dab at random and to cover a large sheet of paper with spots and splodges. When this initial pleasure wears off try printing a blossom tree. Draw a tree trunk, branches and twigs on a large sheet of paper. The child can dab green spots for leaves and pink spots for blossoms. If you stand sufficiently far away from the finished result you might almost imagine a French Impressionist painting!
Some children have great difficulty in following a line

with their eyes moving from left to right as they need to do when they follow a line of print. Spot printing can sometimes help here. Supposing you draw a path across the paper with a house drawn at the right hand side. The child can make footprints from the left hand edge leading to the house. Another popular activity is to make a roadway across the page and print white spots down the middle of it, making sure the child starts at the left hand side. Finish off the picture by cutting out pictures of cars and sticking them on the road.

Making wrapping paper for Christmas or birthday presents is another excellent use for the technique of printing. Perhaps a Christmas tree shape cut from a potato might be used with carrot 'balloons' in between.

For children who want something more difficult than random dab printing, making an all over pattern can be fun, and the finished product makes a good book cover. Fold a piece of paper carefully into well defined squares or oblongs. Open it out flat, and print a shape in the first square. This shape must be repeated in the same position in every other square. The child may perhaps print a circle in the top left hand corner of every square, to be followed by a circle in the centre of each, and then one in the bottom right hand corner. He will find he has made a pattern of spots reaching across the page in sloping lines.

PLAYING WITH LIGHT

Children find great pleasure in lights of all kinds. For proof of this observe their faces as they watch sparklers on 5th November, the fairy lights on the Christmas tree, the night light in the turnip lantern on Hallow E'en, or the candles on the birthday cake. Handicapped children of course share this fascination, and there are some simple ways of using light as a means of attracting their attention and helping them to follow a moving object with their eyes.

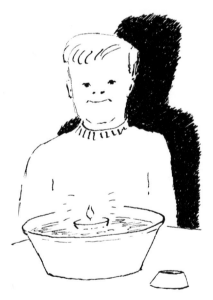

A Torch

This, shone on a baby's hand or the beam moved slowly along the wall nearby, may be a good way of encouraging him to turn his head to follow the spot of light. Two torches can be used to make an excellent

27

hand-eye co-ordination game. Torch Tag was invented by two children who found torches in the toes of their Christmas stockings. The object of the game was for one child to chase with his beam the spot of light created by the beam from the other child's torch. This particular game was fast and furious but it could be equally enjoyable at a slower pace. For the best effect it must be played in the dark of course.

Jack o' Dandies

These are the patterns of light which dance on the ceiling when sunlight is reflected by a mirror or a shiny surface like a knife blade. Less dazzling jack-o'-dandies can be made by putting a bowl of water on a sunny window sill. A slight breeze ruffling the surface of the water will make the jack-o'-dandy dance.

Making shadow Patterns

A bright light shone on a plain wall is all that is needed for this fascinating pastime. Children love to hold their hands in front of the beam of light from a projector while a home movie film show is being prepared, and the same fun can be had with an angle poise lamp or a powerful torch, or even with sunlight shining on a wall. The children hold their hands in the beam of light and twist their hands and fingers into shapes to cast interesting shadows on the wall. They might make a fluttering butterfly or a flying bird, or the shape of a giraffe's head.

Playing with shadows on the ground

In a large play area trying to jump on another child's shadow can be a very good way of using up plenty of energy!

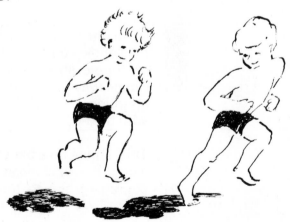

Shadow Puppets

These can be made by hanging up a sheet, holding cardboard shapes quite near to it, and shining a bright light behind them so that a shadow is thrown onto the sheet. If a doorway is used to support the sheet the puppet operator can work in one room while his audience sits in another. Very simple puppets can be made by cutting shapes from old christmas cards and fixing them with sticky tape to pipe cleaners or long strips of cardboard so that the child can control the shape without the shadow of his hand showing on the sheet. Helpful books giving fuller instructions are listed on page 47.

Sun Prints

These take no skill, but quite a lot of patience for they must not be disturbed for several hours. Use a cheap paper which fades in the sun — e.g. poster paper, brown paper or sugar paper. Lay it flat in strong sunlight and arrange on it a cut out shape or a real object such as a sieve or a cheese grater or a piece of wire netting. Fix this so that it cannot be joggled, and after a few hours the paper exposed to the sunlight will have faded, leaving the protected part the original colour.

For Older Children, Making a Floating Candle

Melt down the ends of coloured candles in an old tin, (do not mix up the colours) or add a *small* amount of old wax crayon to white candle wax. Too much crayon will stop the new candle from burning well. Keep all the pieces of wick. Pour the melted wax into a cake patty pan, poke the wick in with a cocktail stick when the wax starts to set and hold it in place for a few moments. When the candle has quite set, turn it out of the mould. Taking care not to get the wick wet, float the candle in a bowl of water and set it alight.

LOOKING AT THE WORLD
A DIFFERENT WAY

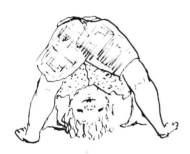

Babies learning to walk discover that they can look through their legs and have an entrancing view of an upside down world. All children like to play tricks with what they see, and the following suggestions may encourage further interesting experiments:-

(a) Peeping through fingers.

(b) Looking down a cardboard tube.

(c) Looking through coloured cellophane from a sweet wrapping or Perspex from a set of Playplax plastic building shapes.

(d) Looking through home-made 'rose tinted spectacles', frames made from pipe cleaners, lenses from coloured cellophane.

(e) Looking through a piece of paper with a hole in it.

(f) Using a magnifying glass or a microscope.

(g) Playing with a mirror. A plastic baby mirror available from many toy shops is double sided and very robust for young children.

(h) Looking through a telescope or binoculars either way round.

(i) Looking through a kaleidoscope.

(j) Looking through an octoscope. This is held in one eye like a kaleidoscope but, instead of seeing a pattern of coloured shapes, the image in front of the octoscope is reflected eight times. This could be a person's face, the view from the window, the child's own hand, etc. Available from some toy shops and department stores.

PUPPETRY

If you have ever watched the expressions on the faces of children enjoying a Punch and Judy Show you will be convinced of the power to attract that puppets can have. Children far too young to be able to make their own puppets love to watch those made by other children, and many older brothers and sisters like to use their imaginations and nimble fingers to make up shows for the younger members of the family. Puppets can sometimes work a sort of magic with shy children and those with speech defects. These children can become so involved in the actions and feelings of a puppet that they can forget their own self-consciousness.

The range of puppetry is very wide. Some figures can be made in a few moments, others are extremely complicated and take considerable skill to manipulate. The following suggestions are for puppets which can be made quickly from scrap materials. If these provide fun and stimulation for your child and start a new interest and you want more information, directions on how to make more elaborate ones can be found in the books recommended on page 47.

Paper bag Puppets

These are literally made in seconds and usually last long enough to provide a lot of fun. Choose a bag without printing on, small enough to fit over the child's fist like a boxing glove. For a cat puppet, for example, the corners can be twisted to make ears, features marked with felt pens, whiskers made out of drinking straws, and the neck gathered in round the child's wrist where it is held in place by a rubber band.

A slightly more durable version of a bag puppet can be made by stuffing the head with a ball of newspaper, and making a neck with a cardboard tube (the inside of a toilet roll or paper towel is ideal). The mouth of the paper bag is gathered round the tube which makes a good firm shape for the child to grip.

Stick puppets

Pop-up dollys on a stick which can play peep-bo from inside their hideout are one example of this kind of puppet. Jack Point in 'Yeoman of the Guard' has his Punchinello to consult, and children often like a simple stick puppet to wave about and talk to. Perhaps the easiest one to make is to convert an old wooden spoon by drawing a face on the back of the bowl with non-toxic felt pens. This puppet has the advantage of being chewable! Other puppets can be made using any stick — a ruler or the handle from an old washing up mop will do — and making a face in cardboard to stick on the top. Extra sophistication can be added by making arms to flap as the stick is twisted. If the hands can be weighted by making them from large buttons firmly stitched on, the arms will swing round with gay abandon! A long skirt can be made by gathering a piece of material round the stick, and the child can hide his hand under its folds. This helps to give the puppet an identity of its own.

Finger Puppets

The very simplest way to make these is by drawing a face on the front of a finger, and wrapping a handkerchief or tissue round it to make a cloak and hood which can be held in place with a rubber band.

More lasting puppets can be made by cutting the fingers from an old white cotton glove and decorating them. Features can be drawn with fibre pen. Wool hair and scraps of material to represent suitable clothing for the character created can be stuck on with fabric adhesive.

Knitted puppets are quite quick to make and grip the finger comfortably. Cast on about 12 stitches in brightly coloured 4 ply wool on No. 10 needles. (This should make a puppet about the right size for a five year old. Adjust the number of stitches, thickness of wool and needles according to the size you want.) Knit about 20 rows in stocking stitch. Break off the wool, leaving a long end attached to the knitting. Thread this through the stitches and pull up tight. Fasten off securely and sew up the side seam. The knitting now looks like a disembodied finger from a glove. Put a little ball of cotton wool (or scraps of cut up old nylon stocking) in the tip to be the head, and wind wool firmly round the puppet just below this to form a neck. Make two French knots in black wool to represent eyes and sew on an orange felt beak. Make another puppet the same way in another colour. Put a finger puppet on each index finger, and you can play the game:

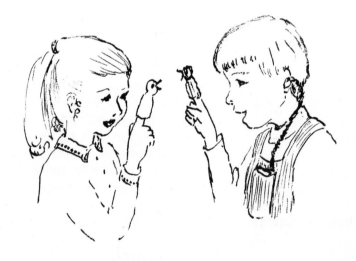

Two little dickey birds sitting on a wall,
One named Peter (show one puppet) the other
named Paul (show the other one).
Fly away Peter (put that puppet behind your back),
Fly away Paul (put the other puppet behind your
back),
Come back Peter (bring him out again),
Come back Paul (ditto with the other).

These knitted puppets can also be dressed in many
ways and finished off to represent different characters.
As they are easy to make it is worthwhile keeping a few
in reserve. They can make a happy diversion for a sick
child, cheer up a hospital visit or provide some fun on an
otherwise boring day.

Non-knitters may prefer to make finger puppets,
simple or elaborate, from felt. This material is ideal as it
does not fray. Seams can be stuck or sewn and the
puppet embellished as required.

Puppets with a Mouth

These can be particularly successful in persuading
reluctant talkers to say a few words.

The simplest ones can be made from an old sock.
Turn in the tip of the toe so that it makes a shape rather
like an egg cup. The depth of the 'egg cup' will depend
on the length of the fingers which will operate the
puppet. The longer the fingers the deeper the
depression needs to be. It is worth while putting a few
stitches along the sides of the foot of the sock to keep
this toe section firmly turned in. To operate this puppet
put all the fingers in the top and the thumb in the
bottom toe pocket. The mouth opens and shuts as the
fingers and thumb are moved apart and together. The
sock can be decorated in many ways. A strip of white
felt cut down the centre with pinking shears will make
fierce teeth for a crocodile or you can add floppy ears
and a lolling tongue to make a different creature.

Chatty Chick

This puppet is particularly good for encouraging speech
and finger and thumb pinching movements because the
beak is made from a hair curl clip which will open and
shut when it is operated from the back of the head. It is
splendid for whiling away long journeys or for amusing

33

CHATTY CHICK

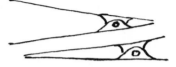

Cut inner shape once in cardboard for stiffening

↑

Hole
↓

Cut outer shape twice in fur fabric. Oversew (right sides together) leaving base open. Turn inside out, insert cardboard and stuff lightly.
Poke "ankles" in the opening and sew in securely. Sew up opening.

A pin curler makes his beak which opens and closes when you squeeze it at the back.

Make a small hole right through the Chick. Poke the beak through from the back to the front. Neaten the back if you wish with a little box of felt. Cover the beak inside and out with orange felt. Stitch firmly to face. Sew on small circles of black felt for eyes, and stitch eyebrows.

Approximate shape of beak covering. This varies according to the size of the pin curler.

Cut 2 in felt

Cut here on one side only. Sew together, round outside edge.

Foot
Cut 4 in felt

Sew two pieces together for each foot.

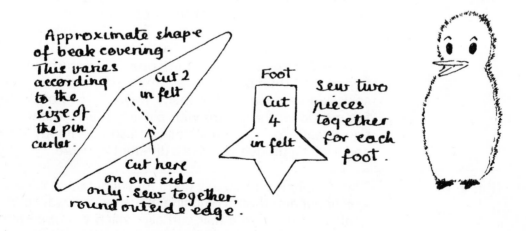

a child in bed. It has been devised by Mrs Olwen Marston of Freshwater (Isle of Wight) Women's Institute.

Glove Puppets

Bought glove puppets are often too large and heavy for small hands, but it is easy for anyone handy with a needle to make one the right size. First cut a paper pattern. Place the child's hand on a piece of paper in the position it will be in when it is working the puppet. Most children like to use their thumb for one arm, their index finger for the neck, their middle finger for the other arm, and the ring and little fingers are tucked into their palm. A few children prefer two fingers to work the head and two fingers for the arm not filled with the thumb. Draw round the child's hand in his chosen position, making a very generous seam allowance. Cut the puppet out in double material and tack round the seams. Try it for size before stitching firmly, and then decorate according to character.

Quickly made glove puppets can be made from Vilene inter-lining. This material (used in dressmaking) is stronger than paper and more pliable. A shape can be cut out, as with a glove puppet, and the seams can be machined or stuck with fabric adhesive. Features can be marked in with felt pen and clothes drawn on. At this stage it is wise to prevent the colour going through to the back of the puppet by slipping a piece of paper inside.

MAKING THE MOST OF JIGSAWS

Some children never really take to jigsaws and this is a pity because puzzles can be such a good way of encouraging careful observation, as well as being fun and a rewarding and peaceful occupation for a child who must sometimes play on his own. Perhaps a dislike first started when a well-meaning adult emptied a box of pieces onto the table and expected the child to make that bewildering muddle into a picture. Many children faced with this situation will avoid criticism and failure by refusing to have anything to do with the puzzle. So it is important to choose a first one that a child can manage without too much trouble. The easiest puzzles are 'inset trays' which are made of two thicknesses of plywood. A simple picture is painted on the top piece and whole shapes of perhaps a tree, or a person, or a house are cut from this. The picture now has holes in it and this piece of plywood is stuck to the bottom piece which then forms a base for the cut out shapes. The child must complete the picture by returning the shapes to their right places. Usually the cut out shapes are fitted with little knobs to help the child to lift them out of the tray. If these are too small for your child to manage they can be replaced by cup hooks or the plastic knobs sold for kitchen cupboard doors.

Slightly more difficult inset puzzles consist of double plywood with the shape of something familiar cut from the top piece. This might be an aeroplane, or a cat perhaps. This shape is then cut into about six pieces and the child must reassemble the shape within the outline on the base board.

It is much more difficult to make an ordinary puzzle with interlocking pieces. In the first place the child must understand that these separate pieces can be arranged to make a picture. The simplest way of explaining this is to show him slowly how it is done! He might be handed the final piece the right way round, to put in the last gap, and he will probably feel he has made the whole puzzle. He might next try putting in all the corner pieces, or those that make up the top row. When he is good at doing bits of puzzle, always finishing the picture, he will know exactly what he is aiming at, and will soon be ready to make the whole puzzle from scratch.

Jigsaw Libraries

If your child is a jigsaw enthusiast it could be worth while enquiring if there is a jigsaw library in your area. Many Toy Libraries have a large jigsaw section and Public Libraries or Social Services Departments may have information on any local scheme. If there is no jigsaw library in your area you might like to join with a few other parents and start one.

In one area a simple scheme is operating. The boxes containing the puzzles are strengthened at the corners with sticky tape and have a label pasted on the base. This cuts out the bother of cataloguing and just gives the number of pieces in the puzzle and its title. It provides a space for all the borrowers to write their names, and for remarks about the puzzle; e.g. whether there are any pieces broken or missing, so that incomplete puzzles can be removed from circulation. The puzzles are delivered to clubs and housebound people who are on the list of the visiting library van.

HOMEMADE TOYS TO ENCOURAGE THE USE OF SIGHT

Mobiles

These are great fun to make and to watch, and can be as simple or as complicated as the creator wishes. They are made to be seen and not touched, so a variety of quite delicate materials can be used. Feathers, silvery paper, sequins, tissue paper—materials such as these which are quite unsuitable for toys that are meant to be handled—may be put to good use and be very pretty to watch. A mobile can even be made from egg shells. These can be painted or left plain, and then suspended from a coat hanger or a lamp shade so that they are like tiny hanging baskets. In each one plant a nasturtium seed in a little damp soil. Remember to water them occasionally and the seeds will germinate and the leaves will dangle over the sides of the egg shells. Ultimately the plants will crack the egg shells and will need to be transplanted in the garden.

Hints on Constructing Mobiles

All materials must be stuck on very securely, and tested before they are hung to make quite sure no trimmings will flutter down onto the child.

Choose imaginative materials, favouring bright colours and glittering ones which will attract attention.

Keep the shapes simple and try to avoid those which look the same even when they rotate. (e.g. Cylindrical shapes.)

Attach to the mobile something that will rattle or rustle for this will also help it to attract a child's attention. Suitable noisemakers might be a string of milk bottle tops, tin lids, tags from cans of fizzy drinks, or streamers of tissue paper.

PLAY HELPS

Display

Use strong thread to suspend the mobile. Nylon fishing line is ideal because of its toughness and unobtrusiveness, but button thread or thin nylon knitting wool will do just as well. Remember to choose a spot where there is a slight draught to make the mobile move, a good light (but not against the glare of a sunny window), and consider the distance the mobile will be from the child's eyes. If he is in bed and it is hung too far away, or too high up he may not be able to see it.

A hook on the end of a metal rod which can be clamped to a piece of furniture is available from Albion (Nursery) Goods Ltd, (see page 153) and this is ideal for hanging mobiles over cots, prams etc.

Coat hangers also make good mobile hangers. The wooden sort can be painted and notches cut at intervals in the top to locate the threads suspending the dangling objects. This stops them from bunching together or falling off. The hanger must also be suspended by a thread so that the whole mobile can move freely.

It is helpful to try to see the mobile from approximately the same position as the child will see it.

A Free-standing Mobile

This kind of mobile is suitable for a child lying on his tummy or side, or for one who cannot see as far as the ceiling. It can make a pretty decoration for a window ledge or locker top. Make it from a wire coat hanger and a yogurt pot which needs to be well weighted. Bend the wire coathanger into an interesting shape and plant it, hook downwards, in the yogurt pot. Fill this up with stones and pour over them some Polyfiller or Plaster of Paris which will soon set and fix the wire shape firmly in the pot. If the mobile is accidentally knocked over it will not matter because the stones cannot fall out. Decorate the pot with felt, scraps of lampshade trimming etc, and hang small objects to dangle from the wire frame.

Simple Mobiles Children Can Make for Each Other

Just hanging up an assortment of objects from a coathanger can make a very attractive mobile. Items suspended might be a foil plate, red transparent packaging from a box of jam tarts, a bunch of gay ribbons or a small toy like an aeroplane.

Treasures Brought Home from a Country Walk

These can make a splendid mobile. Imagine a conker, a few acorns, a large feather and some fluffy Old Man's Beard seeds hanging from a twig. The shapes and colours are beautiful to look at and they also serve as a reminder of the walk. This kind of nature mobile will have a limited life, but this is another point in its favour—the child will not have time to grow so bored with it that he stops looking!

Using Paper Plates

These can be decorated singly, or in pairs glued face to face to give a cushion effect. Perhaps one side can be covered with shiny foil paper to catch the light, and the other decorated with gummed paper shapes, (these may need a dab of strong glue to help them to stick onto a waxy surface), or with felt pen, or possibly a design made from milk bottle tops. A smiley face, made with two circles for eyes and a banana shape for a mouth can look cheerful, and hair can be made from thin strips of rustly paper which will stir in a draught.

Cutting out a Large Shape and Decorating It

Take a piece of shirt cardboard, or the back of a cereal packet, and cut out a large, familiar shape such as a car, a house, or a cat. Remember the shape will rotate in the draught so each surface of the cardboard can be decorated differently, which will make it more interesting to watch. Finding the right position for the thread to suspend a large shape can present problems. Nobody wants to look at a house with subsidence or a car that is for ever going up hill! To overcome this problem a loop of thread can be attached at two points, like a picture cord, and the suspending thread tied to this. The mobile can then be see-sawed on the thread, like a picture on a nail, until it is hanging correctly.

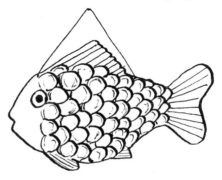

PLAY HELPS

Shapes with a Hole in Them

Children love to cut shapes from the edges of folded paper and then straighten out the folds to see the design they have made. Small sweet papers or the wrappers from chocolate biscuits cut in this way can look very attractive as they revolve, and so can the paper lanterns found in many Infant Schools at Christmas time. To make these, decorate an oblong of paper with a bold design. Fold it in half lengthways so that it now makes a long thin oblong. Cut into the folded edge just over half way, making slits along the whole length of the fold. Open the paper out and bend the shorter ends of the oblong round so that they overlap. Glue them together. Squash the lantern down *gently* from the top so that as it concertinas the slits show up better. Fix a paper handle over the top.

A Family Mobile

This can be made from an old dressmakers' pattern book or from people cut from a magazine. Cut out figures to represent each member of the family. Mount them on plain or shiny paper so that the backs look attractive too, and suspend them from the lamp shade.

A Convection Snake

Cut out a circle of fairly stiff paper about the size of a dinner plate. (Cartridge paper is best, but wallpaper makes a good substitute.) From this make a snake shape by starting at the outside edge and cutting a strip about 1" wide, gradually working towards the centre like the grooves on a gramophone record. Make the final central piece in the shape of a snake's head and trim off the body a little so that the shape becomes thinner towards the end of the tail. Colour both sides of the snake. Make a knot on the end of a length of thread and pass this through the head before tying it to the lamp fitting or hanging it over a radiator. The hot air rising will make the snake twist round. A smaller snake can be made to rest on the point of a pencil stuck into a cotton reel to give it a firm base. This free-standing version works well on a shelf above a radiator, or on the mantlepiece.

Children and parents who want to make more elaborate mobiles will find ideas and much helpful information in the books suggested on p. 47.
Make Your Own Mobiles by T. M. Schegger,

Oak Tree Press   1966
Mobiles Leisure Craft Series
Burns and Oates

Instant Pop-up Dolly

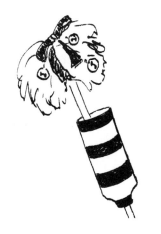

This simple toy, made in a matter of seconds, can give all the excitement and anticipation associated with a real pop-up dolly, which is a doll on a stick and the hem of its skirt is attached to the lip of a cone. As you push the stick through the cone the doll pops up as far as her dress will allow. When the stick is pulled back the doll hides inside her cone. The instant version is made from a detergent bottle and a washing up mop. Cut the base off the plastic bottle and turn it upside down, so that the freshly cut edge is at the top and the neck is pointing downwards. Push the stick of the mop through the upturned bottle and out of the neck so that the mop head is hidden inside the bottle and the stick pokes out of the bottom. By pushing the mop handle up and down you can make the mop head hide, appear, and hide away again. Use a new yellow or red mop with bright ribbon and a budgerigar bell from the pet shop tied on, and baby will enjoy this toy even more. When he is tired of it you can use the mop for its original purpose!

A Transparent Bottle

A rattle made from an empty plastic squash bottle is described in the chapter on hearing (page 67). A plastic bottle can make a splendid looking toy too. The following ideas are all for water filled bottles, and are quite safe to use with younger children. Tough Guys also enjoy them very much, but if they manage to crack the bottles they can make a sloppy mess. Playing with them out of doors or in the bath may be the answer!

(a) Half fill a transparent plastic bottle with water and add a few drops of detergent before firmly screwing on the lid. For a change a few drops of food colouring or powder paint can also be added to make coloured water, or you can use tinted bubble bath. Children enjoy giving the bottle a vigorous shake and then watching the bubbles subside.

(b) Fill a plastic bottle with water and put in some oatmeal or coconut to make a snow storm. The water

41

may become a little cloudy, but the child will not mind. He will be busy shaking the bottle and watching the particles sink to the bottom. When visibility is too bad, empty the bottle and start again!

(c) The best snowstorms are made by filling a small bottle with glycerine and using glitter for the snow. These materials are more expensive but can be suitable for gentle children who need 'low effort' toys.

All these shakers can be useful for children with whom all other toys seem to fail. They have given pleasure to autistic children and to mentally handicapped children too big and strong for shop rattles. They seem to enjoy the feeling of weight as well as seeing the light shining through the bottle and the movement of the 'snow'.

A Swishing Jar

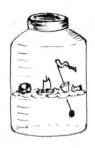

This has proved popular with young partially sighted, mentally handicapped children who are often very difficult to amuse and interest. A large plastic sweet jar, (the kind usually thrown away by confectioners) is needed. Put about three inches of brightly coloured water in the bottom. You can use paint or food colouring to tint the water. Drop small floating objects such as a cotton reel, a wooden bead, a table tennis ball or a cork into the jar. Glue round the edges of the lid and screw it on firmly. Children love to rock the jar and watch the contents bob about.

Scrap Books

These are very personal things when they are made for a particular child and are often much more enjoyed than any bought book. If you have not yet made a scrap book you may find the following hints useful.

(a) Make the subject of your book topical. Children are primarily interested in everything that directly concerns themselves, and a book entitled 'Me' can be a winner! The pages could include photographs of the child and his family, pictures of his favourite toys, a car like the family one, pets, favourite foods, or even the wrapping from a special bar of chocolate brought home from a party. A book like this with direct personal appeal will interest a child far more than the usual kind of scrap book made from a collection of old Christmas Cards.

(b) Keep the book short. A child who enjoys a scrap book may have a very limited span of attention, and perhaps still be at the tearing stage. It is better to spend the time making four thin books than to produce one magnificent fat one. This way the child will have a greater variety of picture books to examine, and should the temptation to tear be too overwhelming it is not as disastrous as the destruction of a large book would be.

(c) Use the strongest and most colourful materials. Wall paper (not the bumpy kind, or the scraps will not stick properly) can be pasted to waste cardboard from cartons, cereal packets or soap powder boxes, to make the pages for an attractive board book. These pages can then be loosely tied together so that they will turn over easily. Another way of making the pages is to cut thick brown paper to a suitable size and stitch the pieces together. Coloured sticky tape can be stuck to the edges of the pages to give them extra strength, and this will also cheer up the brown paper.

(d) Make sure the edges of all the scraps are well stuck down or the temptation to 'pick' will be irresistible!

Care of Scrap Books

If you have taken the trouble to make a special book for your child it will be disappointing if it is soon torn. Look at it together during a quiet moment when you can talk about the pictures, savour and enjoy them. Tearing paper is a most useful and delightful activity with suitable materials at the right time, but a first scrap book should be treated with care. A child will then learn to look upon it as a treasure, and realize that not all paper is for ripping up!

To discourage all but the most determined biters and tearers a scrap book can have each page protected with clear sticky-backed plastic which can be bought by the roll at stationers shops. It is expensive, but a home-made book that has taken time and effort to make may well become a family treasure, and is worth preserving.

A Scrap Sheet

This is just a large sheet of paper fixed to a wall or the back of a door, at the right height for a child to be able to see it properly and to point to the pictures. Every day a new picture can be added until there is no more room.

PLAY HELPS

A Zig-Zag Scrap Book

This makes a change from the conventional scrap book and can be made to stand up so that a child can see all the pictures in a long line. Stiff paper or thin card is folded zig zag fashion so that it can close up and open out like a concertina. Pictures can be stuck on both sides of the zig zag. A good subject for this kind of book could be 'In the Street'. Pictures of cars, lorries, a fire engine, an ambulance, people, bicycles etc could be pasted on each section of the book to be looked at with the book folded or it can be opened out to show a long picture like a frieze.

A Sorting Scrap Book

This kind of book can be particularly helpful to a child with a vocabulary or speech difficulty because it can be a palatable way of practising new or difficult words. Basically it is a large scrap book with only a few pages in it, but each of these has a capacious pocket at the bottom of it. Above the pocket is pasted a picture, and into the pocket go many pictures of objects relevant to the picture. Imagine a young deaf child who is learning the names of objects in his house. His scrap book might have a page with a picture of a kitchen, another with a bedroom or sitting room or dining room, or bathroom etc. Under each picture would be an envelope and into these would go pictures (cut from magazines or mail order catalogues) of articles which would be found in that room—a gas stove, fish slice, frying pan, kettle, for the kitchen; beds, blankets, pillows, sheets, cupboards for the bedroom and so on. The small pictures of objects can be mounted on thin card (postcard or the

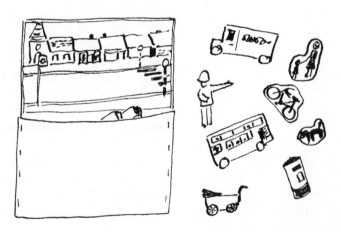

backs of Christmas cards) to make them last longer and if they are to be handled a great deal a covering of transparent plastic film will protect them from grubby fingers. The pockets at the bottom of the pages can be made from the pages themselves by making them extra long and folding up the bottom edge, and sticking it at the sides. Another easy way is to stick on a strong envelope to hold the pictures.

Tracing

This can be an excellent way of encouraging careful looking and hand—eye coordination. Many children find it difficult to hold the tracing paper in place, and clips are not always satisfactory. One certain way of overcoming this difficulty is to buy greaseproof paper sandwich bags sold at most stationers and super-markets. The picture to be traced must be cut a little smaller than the bag so that it will fit inside but will not slide about. Suitable pictures to trace can be cut from old colouring books (jumble sales can be useful here) or you can make your own by cutting out clear, bold pictures and mounting them on stiff paper so that they are the right size to fit the bag. Brothers and sisters often enjoy this job.

A String and Cardboard Spinner

Cut a disc, about 3″ in diameter, from stiff cardboard (or cut several discs from thinner cardboard and stick them together). Decorate with a bold and gaudy design. Faintly draw a line across the widest part of the disc and make two holes, each about 3/4″ (2 cms) from the edge of the disc. Measure two lengths of thin smooth string, each about 2ft long (60 cms). Thread one piece through both holes and join the ends. Thread the other piece from the opposite side and join the ends so that the cardboard disc is now in the centre of two large loops of string. Hold a loop in each hand and flick the disc over many times so that the string becomes tightly twisted. Hold on firmly and pull the hands sharply apart. At the right moment relax slightly, rather like pulling on a chest expander. The disc will rapidly unwind the twisted string and spin on to twist it in the opposite direction. This spinning can be kept going for quite a while once the knack has been learnt.

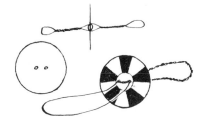

BOOKS TO SHARE WITH CHILDREN

Rag books and board books are the strongest and are easily obtainable from toy and stationers' shops. Ideas for homemade ones can be found on page 43.

Double Colour Books   Perpetua Press 1973
The pages can be covered with a sheet of green or red transparent plastic which will reveal a different picture.

Make a Story Flip Over Books   345 Kiddicraft 1974
Titles include 'In the Country' and 'In the Town'. Each page of pictures is divided into strips on a spiral binding so that an infinite number of scenes can be made.

Macdonald Zero Books for Fun and Learning   1972
These books have clear pictures and give questions on them for the child to answer, encouraging him to have a careful look. Titles include 'In the Jungle', 'In the Garden', 'In the Town', 'In the Air', 'On the Beach' and 'On the Farm'.
Simple text and ideas clearly illustrated. Suitable for *about* seven years and upwards.

Mirror Books   Two titles available from ESA.   See page 153.
'Use the Mirror in this Book'   by Annette
'Make a Bigger Puddle, Make a Smaller Worm' by Marion Walter
Half a picture is drawn and it can be completed by using the unbreakable mirror supplied with the book.

Barnaby Books Titles include 'Learn to Look' and 'Help Yourself Stories'. Strong books with clear pictures. Suggestions on how to use them to the best advantage. Published by Learning Development Aids, Park Works, Norwich Road, Wisbeach, Cambridge PEY3 2AX.

Ladybird Books Particularly the early picture books and the 'Talk About' series. These are especially good for encouraging careful looking.

BOOKS FOR PARENTS AND OLDER CHILDREN

Make Your Own Mobiles
T. M. Schegger   Oak Tree Press   1966

Mobiles
Leisure Craft Series   Burns and Oates

Fun With Puppets and Soft Toys
Valerie Janitch   Kaye and Ward   1974

Puppet People
Starter Activities Series   Macdonald Educational
Plenty of colourful illustrations of easily made puppets.
Simple text suitable for early readers.

How to do Puppetry
Ronald Fairhurst   Nelson
Written to be used by children. Plenty of drawings and simple text. More difficult than 'Puppet People' needing better reading ability and more skill and patience to make the puppets.

Making Easy Puppets
Shari Lewis   Frederick Muller   1967
Recommended for all situations where a quick puppet is needed (e.g. to amuse a sick child, at a party, or for children with a short span of concentration). Many good ideas for making 'instant' puppets from paper bags, match boxes etc and even a carrot! Also includes simple Origami puppets like the fish made from folded paper which opens its mouth when you pull its tail.

The World of Puppets
Lothar Kampmann   Evans
Include patterns for jumping jacks with movable limbs which can be particularly useful for children with limited hand movement, or if made strongly in wood they are. suitable for severely retarded children. Directions for marionettes controlled by strings could interest older children with nimble fingers.

Making and Using Finger Puppets
Margaret Hutchins   Mills and Boon   1973
Strongly recommended for parents and grandparents who like knitting. Finger puppets are devised for many

situations familiar to handicapped children. E.g., a chest of drawers with a puppet in each one—sufficient for the length of a hospital stay. There are also patterns for 'cover ups' for bandaged fingers or toes sticking out of a plaster cast (described as being very good for encouraging a child to 'wiggle'!).

Your Book of Puppetry
Vicki Rutter   Faber and Faber   1969
Written for the more advanced puppeteer. Instructions for glove and string puppets, suitable plays and further reading suggested.

Aquaria
Jim Kelly   Brockhampton Press   1969
How to set up, stock and maintain an indoor fish tank.

Your Book of Bird Watching
Richard Fitter   Blandford Press   1965

The Birds in Your Garden
From the Royal Society for the Protection of Birds, The Lodge, Sandy, Bedfordshire, SG19 2DL.

Keeping Pets
Maxwell Knight and Will Green
Brockhampton Press   1971

Growing Things
Elizabeth Gundry   Piccolo   1974

Indoor Gardening   Ladybird Book No. 633
Look out for other Ladybird Books. They are cheap and sturdy and the list of titles is constantly being enlarged.

Art With Children
Daphne Plaskow   Studio Vista
How parents can provide the right art materials for their child's stage of development. Plenty of illustrations and practical help.

Art and the Handicapped Child
Zaidee Lindsay   Studio Vista

Lots of Fun to Paint
Collette Lamarque   Collins   1973
Plenty of ideas for young artists.

Making Pictures and Patterns
Howard Mell and Eric Fisher
Schofield and Sims   1969

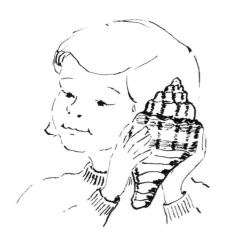

2 Making the most of HEARING

The ideas in this chapter will be helpful to all handicapped children, including sometimes the relatively few profoundly deaf ones who can enjoy and react to the vibrations made by low pitched sounds. Parents of children with some hearing loss know how much they need continuous encouragement and stimulation to make the best possible use of their ears, but all children need to learn to listen and to remember sounds in order to learn to speak. Speech is the quickest and easiest way of communicating with another person, and though it is learnt gradually and without too much effort by most children, some of those for whom this book is written may find it very difficult indeed. Learning to identify noises and to notice what he is hearing will help a child to differentiate between the many sounds which surround him, and in time encourage him to imitate them. A blind child may learn to talk without much trouble but his hearing needs to be developed to a high degree of sensitivity so that it can be useful to him as a mobility guide. The sound of his footsteps on gravel, concrete slabs, grass, carpet, floorboards or vinyl tiles, the special sound of a ticking clock or perhaps the hum of a refrigerator can all help him to pin-point his surroundings. The inflections in another voice, often undetected by us because we can *see* the frown or the smile on the other person's face, may give a blind child a useful clue to the mood of that person. This sort of intensive listening is obviously very important to the many handicapped children who need to use their ears to compensate for another sensory loss, but perhaps most necessary of all is the need to encourage all children to listen so that they can have the maximum amount of *pleasure* from whatever degree of hearing they have.

LEARNING TO LISTEN

Our baby in his pram described in the chapter on sight was combining plenty of listening with his looking. He would hear his mother's footsteps on the garden path, the flapping washing, the birdsong and the bell on his toy. When his mother came to take him in to lunch he would listen to her voice, hear the radio playing, bang his spoon on the tray of his high chair, drop it over the side to hear it clatter on the floor, pat his hands on the tray, clap them together—endlessly experimenting and repeating movements which created sounds and sensations he enjoyed. He would sing through a mouthful of cereal—mum mum mum—and thinking that he was at last saying 'Mum' his mother would reward him with smiles and cuddles, and so perhaps start him off on the road to speech.

In his play he would be creating an endless variety of sounds—patting the plastic chair seat, banging the wooden table, bashing his rattle against the wall, screwing up scrunchy paper—many of these activities he may well have done for the joy of movement and a delicious sense of power and control, but their sound was also part of his pleasure. He would gradually have begun to associate certain sounds with a sequence of events—perhaps a car driving up, a key in the door, and daddy is home; or pots and pans rattling in the kitchen, the chink of metal as the cutlery is placed on the table, or the clatter of a trolley as meal time approaches. The ding dong of the doorbell, the sound of the bath water running in, the noises of family pets, such sounds as these and many more will contribute to baby's idea of home and security.

As he grows he will continue his endless experiments and repetitions. Though he will not realize it he is learning about sounds all the time. One day perhaps he will go to Nursery School or Playgroup and here his listening will be encouraged in many different ways so that sounds will give him even more knowledge and pleasure.

LISTENING FOR THE UNDER FIVES

It is nine o'clock and the children are arriving at Nursery School. There is a cheerful hub-bub as gloves are stuffed into pockets and coats and hats hung on low pegs each with its gay identifying picture. From one of the classrooms comes the sound of the gramophone playing Mendelssohn's A Midsummer Night's Dream Overture. The children in Miss Clarke's class hurry towards the sound and sit quietly in the little ring of chairs listening to the fairy music. Suddenly they hear in the music the sound of a donkey braying and they laugh delightedly, enjoying Miss Clarke's little joke. Yesterday Michael had brought Neddy to school and everyone had admired and stroked this well-loved furry cuddly toy, and had learnt to bray like a donkey. They had taken it in turns to be blindfolded and to try to pin the tail on a donkey Miss Clarke had drawn for them, and they had learnt the Nursery Rhyme

> If I had a donkey and he wouldn't go
> Do you think I'd wallop him? Oh no no!
> I'd put him in a stable and keep him nice and warm
> The best little donkey that ever was born.

Miss Clarke had told them about a real donkey she once knew and they listened attentively to her stories about his naughty ways. Now she plays the donkey music again and the children join in with the eeyores.

Today's big news is centred round the conch shell a sailor uncle has brought home for one of the children. All have a turn at listening to the sound of the sea in the shell. Brian is bored by having to keep quiet while the others listen. He plays with his ear and discovers he can make nearly the same sound by cupping his hand over it. He finds he can make different sea sounds according to the position of his hand, and loudly tells the group of his exciting discovery. They all try it for themselves. Mary runs to the junk box and puts a yogurt pot over her ear, but the result is disappointing. Miss Clarke takes two tins from the junk box and quickly makes a small hole with a skewer in the bottom of each tin. She threads a long piece of smooth string through the holes in the bottom of the tins to join them together, securely knotting the ends so that they will not pull through and with this held taut she shows two children how one can talk into a tin and the sound will carry along the string to

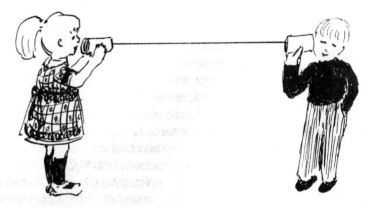

the child listening at the other one. The children soon learn that they must keep the string really tight, but this inevitably becomes a tug of war, and the string pulls out of one tin. Miss Clarke rescues the game by refixing the string and detailing her nursery assistant to hold one tin while she supports the other. Now the children need only to speak or listen, and the crude telephone is working beautifully. Brian decides to make his own telephone with two yogurt pots. He punches holes in the bases but only succeeds in splitting them. He does not know that a hot metal knitting needle is the best tool for making a hole in plastic.

Michael and Mandy have gone to play at the music table. Yesterday Michael discovered that if he chose the chime bars for doh, ray and me he could play 'Mary had a Little Lamb', and he had spent many minutes trying to perfect his performance. Now he wants to repeat his success. Brian comes over to investigate. He knows that if you push a piece of cardboard backwards and forwards under a chime bar you can make the note wobble. They play 'Mary had a Little Lamb' with a wide vibrato, and join in, singing in high pitched falsetto voices with much 'wobble'.

Mandy has noticed an extra long slither box (see Page 71) which Miss Clarke has just made. At first she tips the grit vigorously from one end of the box to the other, enjoying the feeling of the weight of the grit being transferred from one hand to the other, and the sharp slapping sound it makes as it hits the end of the box with force. Her arms begin to tire and she tips the box more slowly, noticing the shooshing whispering sound she is now making. She has heard that sound before. Her face lights up as she remembers that stormy day at the seaside when the waves dashed against the promenade and made that same shooshing sound as they sucked back all the tiny pebbles in the foamy undertoe. Delightedly she runs to share her discovery with Miss Clarke.

Tracy is sad today. She was slow to wake up and the day has turned out all wrong. She has crept beneath the branches of the weeping willow tree that grows in the corner of the play area. She wants to find a hidey-hole where she can be alone and nurse her grievances. A slight breeze flutters the long slender leaves on the dangling branches making a very soft rustling sound. Tracy is soon completely absorbed in watching and listening, her troubles quite forgotten. The breeze dies away for a few moments and the leaves hang limply. Her wonderful soothing secret sound has stopped. The little girl grasps a branch and shakes it vigorously, trying to

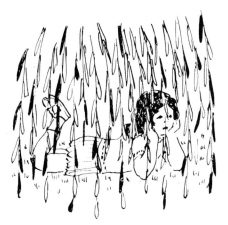

recapture her pleasure. It is not the same. That first magic moment has gone for ever.

Time for lunch. Peter deserts his traffic layout and stops making car noises, Michael stops rushing energetically round the play area where he is whining like a jet and pretending to be the plane that will take him on holiday. Pauline turns away from watching a buzzing bumble bee investigating the flowers; Maureen stops singing to her dolly in the Wendy House; Susan and Sarah leave the window seat where they have been chattering over a familiar picture book, and the children who have been enjoying a percussion band return their instruments to the rack. Soon all are washed and tidy and ready for lunch. They sing 'Thank You for the world so sweet'. Soon all the plates are cleared and some of the children begin to stack them up. One child has just discovered she can push her spoon over her plate in a certain way and produce a hideous ear-splitting noise. She laughs delightedly at the instant reaction of the Nursery Nurse, and repeats the horrible sound twice more before her plate is swiftly removed!

After lunch comes rest time and soon most of the children, used to the regular routine, are fast asleep. Martin is new to the Nursery and he lies awake listening to the muted sounds coming from other parts of the building. The clatter of tin plates being washed up, laughter from the staff dining room, an ambulance hurrying along the street, the budgie in the corner trilling a little song, someone opening a squeaky gate, the sound of a child breathing heavily, the crackle of a page as the Nursery Nurse starts to read a new chapter in her book — he hears all these everyday sounds before he too drops asleep.

So the daily routine of the Nursery School continues. All through the day these children have been making the most of their hearing. They have enjoyed organized sounds like the gramophone record, the tin telephone and the percussion band. They have heard new sounds like the noise of the sea in the shell and the whispering leaves. They experimented with sounds when they played with the chime bars and the slither box and the spoon on the plate. They have imitated mechanical sounds in their traffic play, and throughout the day they have listened to stories and jingles and have talked to each other and the teachers, all the time consolidating and increasing their use of words. Miss Clarke has wisely arranged opportunities for concentrated listening, for quiet times and for plenty of chances to experiment with different sounds. Her practical approach to training children to listen with concentration may well give ideas to parents who want to help their child to use his sense of hearing in new and exciting ways.

MAKING OPPORTUNITIES FOR ATTENTIVE LISTENING AT HOME

For Young Children Try . . .

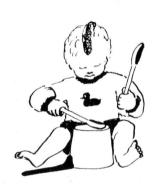

(a) *Providing plenty of noisemakers* for children to shake, bang, kick, hit or drop—sounds which *they* can control. See lists of homemade toys, (page 66) and look around the kitchen for 'instant' percussion instruments. A wooden spoon and an old saucepan or biscuit tin will make a perfect drum, two tough plastic egg cups can be banged together to make a noise like castanets and an old metal spoon stirred round a wire sieve can make a gentle whirring sound.

(b) *Having a code sound* for a certain activity. This might be using a gong or little bell to announce a meal time, splashing a hand in the water before the child is put in the bath, or saying a simple phrase like 'Up you come' before picking baby up. Many of these little traditions can become part of a young child's daily life, adding to his sense of security and making him more aware of his surroundings, particularly if he has not yet learnt many words.

(c) *Speaking to your child* as much as you possibly can. All young babies need to listen to speech for many months before they can sort out and imitate the sounds of words. With handicapped children this listening stage often lasts a very long time and because the child does not appear to respond it can be very easy to forget to talk to him, particularly if he is a 'good' child content to lie placidly where he is put until the next meal time. Finger plays and nursery songs where the child can join in often help to hold a child's attention and there are plenty to choose from in the books suggested on page 74.

For Older and More Able Children Try . . .

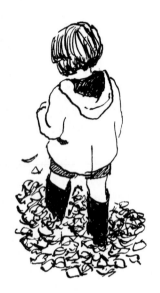

(a) *Going on a 'listening loiter'* (like the 'seeing saunter' on page 13). The object of this sort of walk is not to reach any particular destination but to stop and listen at frequent intervals, staying for as long as necessary at each stop. Sometimes older children like to list the things they can hear, and see how many different sounds they can name. If you listen really hard you will be surprised at how much louder sounds seem to be, and at the enormous number you can identify in quite a short time. It is also fun to use the environment to experiment with sounds. Jumping on a drain cover, scuffing through the Autumn leaves, dragging a stick along a wooden fence or iron railing, blowing on a blade of coarse grass held tightly stretched between the thumbs—what a variety of sounds can be created by even these few activities.

(b) *Listening properly* to the record player, tape recorder, radio or Television. Programmes which ask for audience participation like 'Listen With Mother' or 'Playschool' are excellent for encouraging children to concentrate and really listen. Rationing radio pop music can rescue it from being just a background din, and doing something in time to it, such as playing a simple noisemaker or moving in an appropriate way (jerkily, smoothly etc,) will also help to make it more enjoyable and worthwhile listening to.

(c) *Making sound pictures.* This idea is suggested by Mary Southworth in her book 'How to Make Musical Sounds' (Studio Vista) and can be great fun for a group of children, or for one child with a tape recorder. First think of a situation and then create the appropriate noises which will conjure up that image. An easy one might be 'A Walk Down the Street'. This could include traffic noises, scraps of conversation, footsteps of different speeds to represent young, middle-aged or old people, a Police siren, or special sounds from particular shops, such as music from the Television shop or the chink of wire trolleys and the ringing up of cash tills from the Supermarket. A more difficult sound picture to make might be 'A Walk by the River' with boat noises, ducks, fishermen, lapping water and the rustle of the wind in the reeds. As with painting a picture the subject and complexity of a sound picture will depend on the interests and ability of the child or children creating it.

(d) *Using a Tape Recorder with visual aids.* At Kingston Toy Library we have been experimenting with special tape recordings made for individual children, and each one is on loan with a box of relevant toys and pictures so that the children have an added incentive to listen to the tape.

One such tape was made specially for a slow learner of seven years old who could nearly count to five. It was also enjoyed very much by several young partially hearing children (using their hearing aids to amplify the sound), a partially sighted boy of four, and many 'slow' children with speech and vocabulary problems.

On the Tape	*In the Box*
The rhyme for 'Two little Dicky Birds Sitting on a Wall'	Finger puppets to wear (see page 33 for Rhyme and how to make the puppets.)
The sound of real bird song. Music to move to. 'The Swan' from 'Carnival of the Animals' Saint Saens	
The story of Goldilocks and the three bears.	Characters to act out the story complete with the three different sized bowls of porridge, chairs and beds.
ice 'One, Two, Three'	A budgerigar ladder for the child's fingers to climb.
Child ,, ,, ,, Voice 'Follow me,' Child ,, ,, ,, Voice 'Up the ladder,' Child ,, ,, ,, Voice 'Carefully'. Child ,,	
A marching tune to move to. ('Blaze Away' played by a military band.)	
Rhyme Five currant buns in a baker's shop Big and round with sugar on the top. Along came a boy with a penny one day,	A card giving the recipe for 'play pastry' (see page 148) so that the child could make his own currant buns to buy.

PLAY HELPS

Bought a currant bun and took it away.
(Repeat for four, three, two, and one currant bun.)

A listening game. What time is it?

A clock strikes (not later than five o'clock for this particular tape) and the child must count the number of strokes.

A small gong. The child copies the number of strokes sounded on the tape.

A skipping tune to dance to.
'Girls and Boys Come Out to Play'.

A game for moving. Giant's Steps
The voice on the tape slowly says
'Take two steps . . . one . . . two . . . stop.'
The child takes two large steps, and at 'stop' puts his feet together.
The voice gives other instructions
'Take three steps . . . one . . . two . . . three . . . stop.'
'Take one step . . . one . . . stop.' etc.

'The Blue Danube Waltz', Strauss

A picture of couples dancing in conventional evening dress.

LISTENING GAMES FOR YOUNG CHILDREN

Plink Plonk

This game consists of just dropping a great variety of different articles into an assortment of containers. It can be particularly valuable as a listening game for those children who are not normally in a position to be able to drop their toys to see and hear the effect of this simple action. We all know why mothers attach toys with lengths of ribbon to the sides of cots and prams. The baby who is active and curious will thoroughly enjoy throwing his belongings onto the floor for someone else to retrieve, but the handicapped child may easily miss out on this exciting activity and its social contact. Even if Mum is cross, at least baby feels he is holding her attention! Plink Plonk can be a way of helping even the most severely handicapped child to enjoy the thrill of dropping something and making a predictable sound. As a bonus it gives excellent practice in grasping and letting go, and is an ideal way of presenting a child with

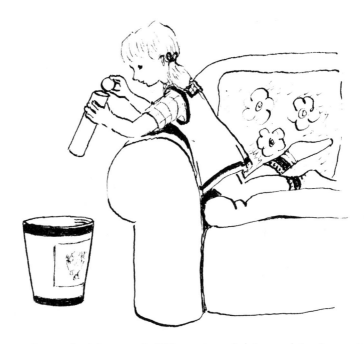

a variety of objects of different weights and textures to feel. Items to drop could include cotton reels, acorns, fir cones, conkers, stones, hair curlers, large buttons or even clothes pegs. Containers to drop them into might be a grocery carton (for a dull thud), a biscuit tin (for a clank), a bucket, plastic or galvanized, or even the kitchen sink! The game can be made more difficult for an older child by giving him a chute to slide the objects down. This encourages him to use both hands and is fun because it makes use of the ever popular activity of posting shapes into holes. The inside of a toilet roll is the simplest tube to manage because of its short length. The inside of a paper towel or oven foil roll can make a slightly bigger challenge for the child, and a long chute can be made from the very strong and heavier cardboard tubes which are used for holding lengths of dress materials, and are thrown away by fabric departments in large stores. When he is using a long tube the child must wait for the dropping noise, and this time lag can encourage him to listen really hard.

Echoes

This can be a good game to play in odd moments or on car journeys etc. It consists of imitating simple sounds like a clock ticking, a fire engine, a car horn, or an animal noise. You make the noise and your child echoes the sound. The noises can be longer and more difficult to imitate as the child learns to listen and remember. It may be possible to let him hear a real echo (perhaps in a valley, between high walls or under a long bridge), and that will really encourage him to listen hard.

Peep Bo

Older brothers and sisters love to play this game with the baby of the family. One hides and says 'Peep peep peep . . .' until the baby is looking in the right direction, and then he bounces out to say 'BO'.

Animal Race Game

This is a game for one or two players and a leader. The players move the animals and the leader must make the noises. A squared surface is needed. This could be a checked table cloth, a tiled floor, a draught board or even some squares drawn on a piece of paper. Put empty tea boxes (or something similar), at one end of the playing area to be the home the animals must make for. Give the child plastic zoo or farm animals which make easily recognizable noises. The child lines the animals up at the edge of the squares and when you make the appropriate sound (e.g. moo like a cow), he can move that animal one square nearer to its home. To make a change you could use 'animal cries' to make the sounds. These are available at many toy shops and consist of a cardboard cylinder contining a noisemaker. When the cylinder is inverted it makes the noise of a cow, sheep or cat.

Start-Stop Games

Like Musical Bumps and all its variations these games are based on moving to a sound and stopping when it ceases. Noises to move to could be music from the radio or record player or piano, bells shaken, a note hummed, a shaker rattled etc. A child who finds movement difficult can shake a waver made from thin strips of coloured paper tied or Sellotaped to an old toilet roll spool or a short length of stick. Another child might like to make his fingers dance or lightly clap his hands, or rub two sandpaper blocks together. It is important that the activity should be a fairly quiet one, and not so attractive that the child is so busy doing it that he forgets to listen for the noise to stop!

Musical Chairs

Have a chair for each child. Arrange these either in a circle with a space between each, or in a line with alternate chairs facing in opposite directions. Before the game begins remove one chair so that one child must stand up. When the music begins the children walk round the chairs. When it suddenly stops they must all try to sit down. The child now left standing is 'out'. Another chair is removed and the game continues until two children are competing for one chair and this decides the winner.

Musical Hats

The children stand in a circle facing the back of the child in front. All but one must wear a hat. When the music plays they pass the hat to the child behind and take a hat from the child in front. When the music stops the child not wearing a hat is 'out'. There must always be one hat short, so at each pause one must be withdrawn.

Musical Mats

The children run round in a circle, jumping over a mat at one place. When the music stops, the last child over the mat is 'out'.

LISTENING GAMES FOR GROUPS OF OLDER CHILDREN

Giant's Treasure

The giant sits in the middle of the room, guarding his treasure which is a little bell, or other noisemaker. He is blindfolded. The children sit in a large circle round him. When given a signal by the organizer of the game one child must try to creep forward and steal the giant's treasure. If the giant hears him coming he must point in the direction of the sound. If he points correctly, the thieving child must return to his place. For children with a slight hearing loss the game can be adapted by giving the thieving child some percussion bells to carry.

The Bell Game

This game has obvious hazards and must be well supervised and played in an unobstructed space, but for energetic older children it can be great fun. All the children but one are blindfolded, and given a whacker made out of rolled up newspaper. The odd child has bells hung round his neck, waist, wrists, ankles, — wherever convenient. He must then dodge between the whackers and try to get from one end of the play area to the other.

Grandmother's Footsteps One child is Grandmother, and stands at one end of the room, facing the wall. The rest of the children stand with their backs to the opposite wall. When the game begins they must creep forward and try to touch Grandmother. If she hears a sound she can turn round. If she *sees* a child move she can send him back to the start. This game needs firm refereeing or heated arguments can arise! It is always a favourite though, and encourages concentration and balance in the children and acute listening by the Grandmother. For the sake of this last virtue it is best played in a large room.

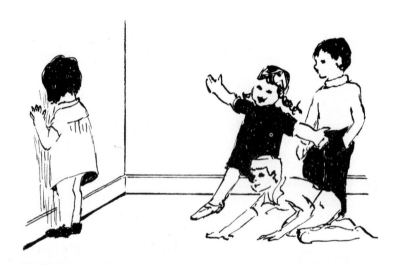

The Ring Master One child is blindfolded and stands in the centre of a circle of children. They dance round him until he cries 'Stop'. He points to someone in the circle and says 'Make the noise of a lion' (or horse, cat, mouse, dog etc.). He must try to guess which child is making the noise.

Traffic Lights This is one of many such games which involve careful listening to directions. If the leader calls out 'Red' the children must sit down, for 'Amber' they must stand still and for 'Green' they must run about.

Do This, Do That

This is a less lively 'directions' game than Traffic Lights. The children imitate simple actions like standing on one leg, pointing to the ceiling or clapping. They must only do the action if the leader first says 'Do this'. If he says 'Do that' they must continue to do the previous action.

Simon Says

This is played like the game above, but the child must only do the action if Simon says so. E.g. 'Simon Says clap your hands . . . Point to the floor.' The children must continue to clap their hands because Simon did not say 'Point to the floor.' Both these games can be enjoyed by children in bed, or by those who find running about games impossible.

Animal Treasure Hunt

The children are divided into teams, each represented by a noisy animal. Rice, or butter beans (which are easier to find) are hidden all round the room. The children each find a bean, but they may not touch it. They make their animal noise in front of the bean to attract the attention of their team leader who is the only one who may collect it. When this has been done the child runs off to find another bean. The winning team is the one with the biggest collection of beans. This is a very noisy game and best played with a large group of children.

Spinning the Trencher

If played with a tin plate this game can be fun for blind children as well as for those with sight. Everyone sits in a circle and each is given a different number. The leader spins the plate and might call out 'Two'. The child whose number that is (perhaps guided by the sound of the spinning plate), must rush towards it and try to catch it before it topples over. If he succeeds, everyone claps. In any case he returns to his place and listens for his number to be called again.

MAKING MUSIC

For suggestions for creating cheap noisemakers see the section on homemade instruments, page 67.

PLAY HELPS

Musical Instruments

For serious music making all instruments must be of a good quality. A cheap instrument may be impossible to tune properly, and is unlikely to produce a satisfactory tone. Making music can be a challenging and enriching hobby for any child blessed with a 'good ear', and for a handicapped child, learning a suitable instrument and being able to play it well can give him much happiness and lead to the forming of many new friendships.

The following firms will send catalogues illustrating the wide variety of orchestral instruments they can supply, also information on Carl Orff percussion instruments which are particularly strong and well made:

Educational Supply Association,
Pinnacles,
P.O. Box 22,
Harlow,
Essex CM19 5AY

London Music Shop,
218 Great Portland Street,
London, W1N 6JH

Playing a Recorder

Many children find great pleasure in playing recorders or guitars. These are more reasonably priced than orchestral instruments like violins and oboes and can be best for a beginner. Quite a high standard can be achieved in a comparatively short time. Here are a few guide lines to help parents who feel their child would enjoy making music but do not know how to start him off.

For able children who have good hand control and whose fingers are physically large enough to cover the holes on the instrument efficiently, playing a Recorder is an excellent introduction to skilled music making. Recorders have many advantages as an introductory instrument.

(a) They are cheap.
(b) They are easily obtainable in wood or plastic.
(c) They are small and portable.
(d) They are virtually unbreakable.
(e) They are capable of being played really well in a reasonably short time.
(f) They give a good introduction to musical notation. The range is not too wide and only one clef is used.
(g) Having mastered the treble recorder—the usual

school instrument—enthusiasts can then learn the descant, tenor or bass recorders. Some families learn to play all these between them, and then are able to enjoy the wide range of music available, and give pleasure to others by their high standard of performance.

(h) There is a wealth of music obtainable at many Public Libraries and local music shops, or from

Schott and Co Ltd,
48 Great Marlborough Street,
London, W1

who also publish 'Recorder and Music Magazine' four times annually.

'Your Book of the Recorder' by John M. Thomson, published by Faber and Faber, is an excellent book which gives information about the four types of recorder and the range of each. It gives advice on how to learn to play and suggests Tutors for teaching yourself. It also lists music available for different stages of proficiency.

Making and Playing Bamboo Pipes

(Suitable for older dextrous children.) These are simpler to play than recorders because the fingering of the holes is easier. Once the mouthpiece has been made and the 'window' cut it is comparatively easy to file out the holes until each note is in tune. Children can learn to play little rhythms and tunes, making these more complicated as each new hole is added. 'Making and Playing Bamboo Pipes' by Margaret Galloway gives all the information needed, and can be obtained from Dryads, Leicester. This firm also supplies tools. Bamboo can be obtained from carpet shops and interior decorating specialists where it is sold for curtain rods.

Playing the Guitar

The guitar is another instrument which can be played with reasonable efficiency and much enjoyment within a comparatively short time. It is cheaper than other stringed instruments and a child with a 'good ear' who can remember tunes and harmonies easily can soon play well enough to give himself and others a great deal of pleasure. A guitar is reasonably light and portable and makes a gentle sound not too annoying for the neighbours! It is also the most popular instrument of our time among teenagers and can be a very successful means of helping a young handicapped person to integrate with others of his own age.

There are many simple tutors available, including 'Play Guitar' by Ulf Goran (in association with Yorkshire Television) published by the Oxford University Press. This one is suggested for several reasons. It assumes a complete lack of musical training, and really begins at the beginning. It incorporates a gramophone record showing how many of the tunes should sound, and playing with this makes the early stages much more interesting. The tutor is illustrated by a cartoon character called Floppy. The whole approach is light hearted and may well suit a teenager whose left hand is large enough to stretch the distances required to make the notes, and who has sufficient persistence to puzzle out the instructions. Suggestions are also made for using simple percussion instruments which can be played by other members of the family. Industrious pupils can progress to 'Play Guitar 2' and 'Play Together—for Voice and Guitars' both by Ulf Goran.

BOUGHT MOBILES WHICH MAKE SOUNDS

Musical Mobiles or Wind Chimes

These are designed to be hung out of reach, and like ordinary mobiles they are restful and pleasant to watch. They also make a gentle sound which many children find very attractive. Some are made from strips of coloured glass, others from wood or metal, and when the draught catches them they produce a soft tinkling sound. Large stores sell 'Angel Chimes' at Christmas, and these must be placed where they can be seen and heard, but not touched. Four lighted candles cause a draught which turns a fan. Four Angels hang from this, and dangle metal rods which strike little bells as the fan revolves. Shell Wind Chimes are sold at some Oxfam shops.

HOMEMADE NOISEMAKERS

All these can be made from odds and ends, and can be

adapted to be just right for any particular child. Some can be played with one hand, others encourage the use of two. Some are good for breath control while others can be enjoyed by children with very little physical movement. All children like to make a noise, and feel a satisfactory sense of power if they can control the sounds they create. Used more skilfully, as in a band, or being played in time to the radio, these simple instruments can be very helpful in encouraging concentration, co-ordination and listening hard.

Rattles

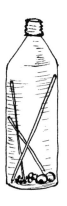

(a) *From a Plastic Fruit Juice Bottle.* Make sure the bottle is clean and dry, or the contents may stick to the sides which can also become clouded with condensation. Any filling may be used, but for a really determined child who might manage to open the bottle it is sensible to use edible things like a few long sticks of spaghetti, dried peas, lentils or rice. For a gentle child it can be quite safe to use buttons, beads and strips of shiny paper or baking foil. These look more attractive and may make a slightly louder noise. When the contents are inside the bottle the lid must be firmly fixed on with a little polystyrene cement. This rattle is ideal for a gentle child and for the very young. Its size and light weight and the visibility of the contents as it is shaken about make it very appealing. It is not suitable for strong children who might crush and shatter the bottle.

(b) *From a Detergent Bottle.* This is much more robust than the rattle above and will stand a heavier filling such as small stones. The stopper must be glued on securely and the plastic loop which normally keeps the stopper closed must be cut off in case it is chewed. The outside can be made more attractive if the printing is scrubbed off with wire wool and the bottle painted with Humbrol Enamel (obtainable in small tins and really intended for painting plastic models.) This paint is lead free and quick drying and can transform this rattle into a special toy instead of just the disposable container it really is.

(c) *From an inverted treacle tin.* This rattle resembles a crude ship's bell. It is suspended by its handle, and the

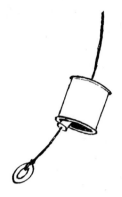

child shakes the clapper inside. It is specially good for 'throwers' and 'droppers' because it must be hung up. Take the lid off the tin and punch a hole in the middle of the base. (Push from the outside inwards so that the rough edges are inside.) Thread a piece of thick white string, about 18" long, through the hole—piping cord is splendid for this job because it looks attractive and is soft to feel. Make a loop in the string outside the base of the tin. This is used to hang the rattle up by. Make a knot inside the tin to stop the string pulling through and thread on a cotton reel which will be used to knock against the sides of the tin like a clapper of a bell. Tie knots to hold this reel in position, and tie another cotton reel or a large ring to the end of the string for the child to grasp. Paint the tin and hang it up so that he can reach it easily.

(d) *A very loud rattle from a small tin.* Choose a stout tin such as one used for cough sweets, toffees or floor polish. Use at least two screws to attach the handle to the lid. (An odd cylindrical building brick makes an excellent large shape to hold.) A dab of very strong adhesive fixes the handle even more firmly. Put in small stones or ball bearings (discarded rusty Bagatelle balls are excellent) small bells from a pet shop or even nails if you have faith in your ability to fix the lid so that it is absolutely child proof! Araldite metal adhesive round the rim should make a very secure bond. This is a lovely loud, robust rattle for young deaf children and some older slow learners who still need this kind of toy although they are too strong for the normal babies' rattles, but a word of warning. It could also be a most efficient 'clobber stick' if used, unsupervised, by rough children.

(e) *From small pieces of junk which will jangle together.* This rattle is quick to make and can either be held in the hand or hung up for a child to hit or kick. Suitable metal or hard plastic objects like bottle tops without sharp edges, film spools, Elastoplast spools, or even large buttons are threaded onto sturdy wire (sharp ends must be protected) or string, which can be shaken about to make the threaded objects dance and jingle. A good hand grip can be made from a bicycle handle bar grip.

(f) *A jingle thumper from a broom stick and metal bottle tops.* This noise maker is intended to be held vertically and banged on the floor. It makes a satisfying thump and jingle, and has been adapted for a severely Spastic child by suspending it near her chair with a piece of elastic. She was able to grasp it with one hand and pump it up and down, rather like tolling a bell.

(g) *From Papier Mâché.* Rattles made this way are slower to construct but can be worth the extra effort. They are very strong and colourful when they are finished. This is a good technique for making large rattles for older children. Choose any suitable container such as a margarine tub, a Yogurt pot, a cardboard box or even a partially inflated balloon. Put in the filling to make the rattle. This could be a few peas (dried!) or rice, or pebbles, or a bell. The paper covering will muffle the sound a little, so do some experimenting to make sure that the rattle will make a satisfactory noise. Make a handle from the cardboard cylinder from a toilet roll or a paper towel, or a roll of paper, or with cotton reels glued together. Fix this to the rattle by long narrow strips of paper stuck firmly to both the handle and the rattle. It may be necessary to leave the first layers to dry and then add plenty more until the handle is fixed really firmly. The larger and heavier the rattle the longer this will take. Then cover the entire rattle and handle with *at least* eight layers of pasted paper. It is helpful to use newspaper for one layer, coloured paper for the next, then back to newspaper, and so on. By using different colours for each layer the whole rattle can be covered evenly and there will be no thin places. When the rattle is strong enough and quite dry it can be covered with emulsion paint to hide the newsprint, and then painted gaily with Humbrol enamel.

Rattles in Pairs to make a Sound Matching Game

Collect an even number of identical containers with lids—detergent bottles, plastic pots with lids (such as those used to hold potato salad etc in delicatessen shops,) drug tins—all these are suitable. Whatever you use it is essential that the containers should all be identical and the contents invisible. Arrange the pots in pairs, and fill each pair with the same substance before glueing on the lids. The aim of the game is to shake the pots until the two making the same sound can be put together. Suitable fillings for the containers might be rice, dried peas, butter beans, grit, pebbles, coins, bells, buttons, sand, nails or bottle tops. It is important that the weight of the pots should be as nearly the same as possible, and that the pairs of sounds are clearly distinguishable from each other. Rice and lentils shaken in the same sort of container can sound very similar, so there is need to experiment here. The size and material of the container will alter the sound made by the various fillings. To make sure these shake easily it may be necessary to make a very small hole in the container to equalize the atmospheric pressure. This can be done easily with a hot sewing needle held in a cork.

A Drum

The best possible 'instant' drum is made from an upturned saucepan or an old biscuit tin, with a couple of wooden spoons for beaters. More sophisticated ones can be made by tightly stretching a piece of rubber inner tube over a suitable tin, but there are various snags for the inexperienced. The rubber needs to be reinforced round the edge to prevent it from splitting when it is stretched, and the tension must be applied gently and evenly all round. This can either be done by having inner tube over both ends of the tin like a bongo drum and lacing the drumheads together with a thread which zig zags between them, or if only one drum head is wanted a ring can be held under the base of the drum and the thread passed through this each time.

Clappers

These can be made from any two pieces of wood about the size of the base of a date box. A cotton reel glued on makes a good handle.

Gong

Any strong metal article which can be suspended can be used as a gong. Perhaps an old frying pan, or a horse shoe, or a large saucepan lid might do. At the Adventure Playground at Chelsea there is a row of metal tubes hanging from a bar. Children like to run along the row, drawing a stick across the tubes, making a gorgeous clatter like dragging a stick along a fence—only better!

Scraper

This can be made from any firm material with a ridged surface. A block of wood with ridges filed in it, an old fashioned wash board, fluted pelmet board, ridgy metal doorstep protector, even fluted cardboard are all suitable. Rub the ridged surface with a stick or let the child wear thimbles on his fingers. As well as giving him a close affinity with the sound he is creating he gets a delightful tingling sensation through his fingers.

Happy Hummer

This is a fragile noisemaker, but fun while it lasts. Find a cardboard tube from an empty toilet roll. Fix a piece of waxed paper (from the inside of a cereal packet) over one end with a rubber band. Make a small hole in the side of the tube just above the paper. The child hums into the open end of the tube and the waxed paper should vibrate, making a buzzing sound rather like blowing on tissue paper over a comb. There is a knack In getting the hummer to work properly and experimentation is necessary!

A Slither Box

This is made like the papier mâché rattles, but it is easier to construct as it has no handle to fix. Use a fairly large flat box such as a soap powder box, a chocolate box or a cereal packet. Put in a few spoonfuls of gravel, or grit sold for aquaria, or rice or dried peas etc., according to the kind of sound you wish to make. Cover the box with papier mâché and finish off as described for the rattles. Slither Boxes with grit inside can be particularly successful because children love the feeling of the weight being transferred from one hand to the other as they tip the box and the grit slithers down.

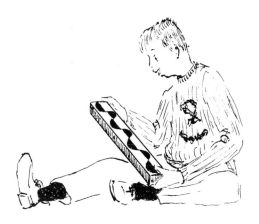

Noisy Busy Board

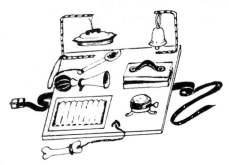

Suitable noisemakers can be screwed to a conveniently large piece of wood. These might include a bicycle bell, a large staple with a budgeriegar bell threaded on it which can be flicked over the curve of the staple from one side to the other, a strip of ridged doorstep protector with a large blunted nail attached by a piece of string conveniently near by to rub across the ridges, or a horn with a bulb to press. Ingenious fathers can devise battery operated bells or a type of Morse buzzer. There are plenty of other ideas many of which make a noise, in 'For Busy Hands' available from the Toy Libraries' Association.

A Soap Box Pull Along

Save a strong packet such as one which has contained washing powder. Punch a hole in the middle of the top and bottom. Thread a piece of string about one yard long through both the holes, going in one and out of the other. Tie a cotton reel firmly to each end of the string to prevent it from being pulled through the box. Put a few pieces of macaroni or pebbles inside; enough to make a good sound. Sellotape the box together to make it really strong. This sort of pull-along is suitable for indoor use by the not too energetic, and many toddlers are fascinated by the way the string disappears into the box and comes out the other side. They will spend considerable time pulling alternate cotton reels. For garden use a covering of Fablon will considerably lengthen the life of the box.

A Clanky

(See also under 'Threading Anything' in the chapter on Touch, p. 94.)
Just thread together the noisiest junk you can

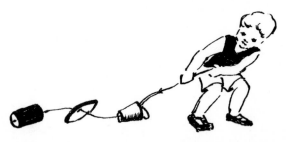

find—perhaps an old tin cup, a bent spoon, and an old saucepan lid, and when the neighbours are out let your toddler rush up and down the concrete path dragging this behind him! (This toy is not suitable for group play where it might get tangled up in other children's legs.)

A Roller Rattle

Use a 2lb treacle tin, punch a hole in the middle of the top and bottom (punching inwards to avoid sharp edges,) and thread a piece of thick string about 1½ yds long, through both holes. Tie the ends together so that the knot will be inside the tin. Put in some stones and fix the lid on firmly. The child can have fun pulling the roller rattle along by the string handle.

BOOK LIST

Music for the Handicapped Child Juliette Alvin   OUP 1965

Playing Instruments
They can Make Music Philip Bailey   OUP
Making and Playing Bamboo Pipes Margaret Galloway   Dryad
Your Book of the Recorder John M. Thomson and Faber   1968
Play Guitar Ulf Goran   OUP   1974
Selmer 'Play it Easy' Tape Learning Courses for the Trumpet, Trombone, Clarinet, Saxophone, Flute, Percussion, Guitar etc. Details from Henri Selmer and Co Ltd, Woolpack Lane, Braintree, Essex. CM7 6BB
The Young Person's Guide to Playing the Piano Sidney Harrison   Faber and Faber   1973
(For talented young pianists.)
Sounds and Music   Macdonald First Library   1974
How music is produced by wind, string and percussion instruments.

Homemade Instruments
Make Music Fun   Avril Dankwork   Dryad
Making Musical Instruments Peter Williams   Mills and Boon (A set of instruction cards.)
How to Make Musical Sounds Mary Southworth Studio Vista

Books of Jingles, Finger Plays and Nursery Songs
This Little Puffin   Compiled by E. Matterson   Penguin
All Sorts of Everything   Malcolm Carrick   Heinemann
The Oxford Nursery Song Book   Compiled by Percy Buck   OUP   1961
The Faber Book of Children's Songs   Donald Mitchell and Cary Blyton   Faber and Faber   1970
30 Songs for Nursery and Infant Schools   Boosey and Hawkes
20 Singing Activities for Tinies   Evans

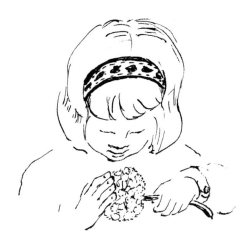

3 Making the most of TOUCH

The purpose of this chapter is to suggest ways in which all children can 'use their sense of touch for pleasure, and for the encouragement of their all round development by learning to be more aware of what they feel. The toys and activities suggested help to make hands controlled and skilful and many will introduce children to new textures and 'feely' experiences. The following pages should be particularly useful for blind and many physically handicapped and chair-bound children.

THE IMPORTANCE OF LEARNING TO TOUCH

For blind children the senses of touch and hearing must obviously be developed to their fullest potential to compensate for the loss of sight. For the purely practical requirements of daily living this must be so. E.g. the little girl with sensitive finger tips can sort her nylon socks into pairs even if the patterns on the legs of each pair are different. Gloves can be worn more easily if the position of the thumb is in the right place to start with, and even tights can be put on with less of a battle if the gusset for the heel is sorted out first. Recognizing toys by their feel or identifying parts of a room by touching the textured wallpaper, or the cold kitchen tiles, or the moquette of a particular chair cover, are a few ways the young blind child uses his hands to

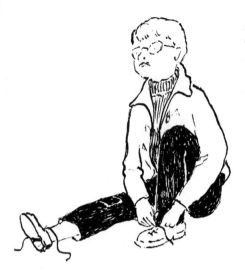

achieve some independence. This is one way he learns to orientate himself to his own environment. He will gradually discover how to undress and dress himself, managing buttons, laces, zips, hooks and poppers; he will go shopping, sorting and counting the coins he needs; he will run errands finding his way about by feeling for familiar landmarks and he will learn Braille. For this he will need not only a good memory but also very sensitive finger tips to help him distinguish between the various combinations of the six tiny dots which make up the Braille symbols. Such sensitivity in the finger tips can be encouraged by playing games such as Feely Bingo or Feely Dominoes (described in the section on Homemade Toys, page 111, which were specially designed to help a newly-blinded child learn to sort and match a wide variety of textures. They helped to develop this essential sensitivity of her finger tips so that she could confidently identify the different feels. The skill she acquired through these games helped a great deal when she began to learn Braille.

A child who needs to spend long hours in one place because his legs are his handicap, will find that if he can train his hands to be nimble and creative he will have at his disposal many more ways of enjoying himself during his leisure time. By developing his hand control and increasing the sensitivity of his fingers through a variety of toys and activities when he is young, he might even train himself to achieve the kind of professional dexterity needed by such people as musicians, or watchmakers.

Sometimes a slow learner or a withdrawn child may need a great deal of encouragement even to perform such simple movements as holding and releasing. Many such children can be persuaded to use their hands if the 'reward' is sufficiently enticing. Perhaps a child who enjoys a music box may consent to pull the string to wind it up. If he likes surprises he might press the button on the Pop-up-Cone-Tree, (a spring loaded toy which 'explodes' dramatically when a child presses the knob to release the spring), or play with a Jack-in-the-Box. With these toys he has been rewarded because of the effort he has made with his hands.

At the other end of the scale is the child who clumsily

grabs at everything he can reach, managing to destroy most of it. Here the problem is not how to encourage him to touch, but how to help him to do it in a less destructive way. It is a very difficult problem to cope with, (particularly if the destructive child is also a 'thrower'), but the longer it is left untackled the larger and stronger the child will become. The 'loving and caring adult' will find, as many parents have, that a little time spent playing *with* a destructive young child can often be of great benefit to him and incidentally to the whole family. A tough two year old should be able to play happily with large strong toys designed for his five year old brother. If he is being played with, shown what to do with the chosen toy (other than destroy it!) and he can share the enjoyment of his play, the tendency to throw can often be forestalled. With luck he may outgrow it, or possibly channel it into a more socially acceptable skill by becoming a champion at skittles or bowls!

Fingers can be compared with tentacles or feelers. They give us an enormous amount of information which experience teaches us to interpret. Hot, cold, heavy, light, big, little, hard, soft. Once we have understood the meaning of such words these are just some of the comparisons we can make instantly with our hands. We can grasp, screw, pull, poke, twist, squeeze and pick up tiny things. Most important of all, we can use our hands to hold tools. As adults we often ignore the value of our hands until perhaps an accident suddenly makes them unusable. Without the help of our fingers we are unable to clothe, feed or clean ourselves and leisure time stretches out into a seeming eternity of boredom. With only one hand functioning normally it is possible to be completely independent of other people but with both hands in working order every desired activity may be literally within reach.

LEARNING TO TOUCH

At a very early age all babies start to discover the world with their fingers. At first they grope and clutch—perhaps clinging on to Dad's finger with astonishing strength or turning their tiny hands round in a blanket and filling all the creases between their fingers with fluff. They discover they can suck a fist or a thumb and with this elementary and conscious movement of carrying something to their sensitive mouths they begin to discover what is pleasant to suck and what is not. The baby in earlier chapters lying in his pram in the garden could use his fingers to explore everything within reach—his fluffy woollen ball, the plastic side of his pram, his own fingers and toes. When his Mother picked him up he would pat the soft skin on her face, twine his fingers through her hair and try to carry her necklace to his mouth for further exploration. When he could sit up he learnt to stretch forward and sideways to try and touch things tantalizingly just out of reach. When he wanted a favourite toy (or the twitching end of the cat's tail) badly enough he learnt to 'swim' and finally crawl across the floor to reach it. This opened up

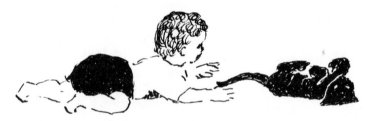

a new world full of a rich variety of stimulating textures, including hard table legs, soft fringes on rugs, cold smooth lino and other exciting things like colourful magazines on low shelves.

The real breakthrough for his busy fingers would come when he learnt to stand at a chair and play on a flat surface uncluttered by his legs. He could reach for more things, open cupboards, take off lids, pull things down on himself and during his waking hours send his Mother nearly distracted by all this endless activity. Of course there were still many disadvantages. In this exciting new world he was likely to be grabbed firmly round the middle at any moment and be whisked away from some absorbing investigation.

His image of adults was often limited to a good view of their hemline and knees. Learning to climb altered even this and he could soon manage stairs. Sitting

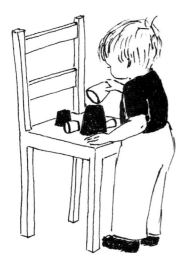

halfway up he would have a birds' eye view of life downstairs. He could climb on a chair and reach further and further, his busy fingers never still. His Mother would complain that he was 'into everything' and gradually the ornaments, pot plants, sewing box and all things fragile or dangerous would be shut away or put on higher and higher shelves. This instinct to feel, to learn through our fingers, and to enjoy the sensations of touching, seems to last us all our lives. Even as adults enjoying the exhibits in a museum or art exhibition or wandering round a department store, we are often faced with notices saying 'Please do not touch'.

LEARNING TO TOUCH IN A ·SPECIAL SCHOOL

Making use of textures

Developing an awareness of textures is one sure way to encourage busy fingers to become more sensitive. Recently I visited a unit for children who were deaf, blind or partially sighted and mentally handicapped. They were between $2\frac{1}{2}$ and 5 years old. All had a different amount of hearing, sight and intelligence but restless hands were common to them all. Making use of the sense of touch was obviously the best way of helping these children to develop confidence, curiosity and some degree of concentration. Later on they might be taught to communicate with hand signs.

The activities and environment devised by their teachers may suggest ways in which parents could also make a child's surroundings more stimulating to his sense of touch.

The school room was part of a special unit attached to a First School. It was opposite the toilets and washbasins and part of it was partitioned off to make a tiny kitchen, and a small room where children could receive individual help. Low pegs were on the wall in the corridor outside, each with the usual shoe rack and low seat. Because of the childrens' multiple handicaps, their pegs were labelled with large raised symbols—similar to the little pictures one associates with all nursery school pegs—but these could be recognized by touch, and were about 3″ square. One was of a raised butterfly moulded in Polyfilla, with buttons imbedded in the wings to represent the spots. Another, for a partially-sighted child was a large letter P cut from a polystyrene tile covered in baking foil and mounted on a sheet of shiny pink card.

Inside the classroom the use of the sense of touch was perpetually encouraged. Parts of the floor were Marley tiled, others were carpeted so that even with their feet the children could know their position in the room. The tops of the cupboards were covered wth strips of carpet samples and one was decorated with imitation grass given by a friendly greengrocer. Hanging from elastic just above a work table, within easy reach of the children, was a large mobile. It had ladybirds made from egg boxes with pipe cleaner legs which could be bent in different directions, and a cardboard fish with crunchy paper stuck each side to give him a fatter shape. Part of the floor — the carpeted area — was used for floor games and at the edge of this part of the room was hung a large hessian sack filled with sweet-smelling hay. It was suspended by a spring so that it could be made to bob up and down with very little exertion and was completely harmless if a child happened to bump into it. Attached to it were strings of bells, a Rupert Bear, patches of sponge rubber to pick off, a string of chunky beads and some strips of cellophane packing paper. Across one corner of this area was slung a hammock, a few inches from the floor. The children could nearly all manage to get themselves on and off and if they misjudged the distance the soft carpet cushioned their fall. Other favourite toys were a large brightly coloured vinyl beach ball from a chain store (costing about 60p) and an old car inner tube which presumably cost the Unit nothing. A row of low shelves held the childrens' table top toys and acted as a room divider, making a little bay where there was a special work table. This was square and larger than the usual nursery school table. In the centre of each side was a scooped out semi-circle where a child could stand with a small gate fastened behind him to keep him secure. The teachers found this table ideal for helping the children to concentrate on whatever toy they were playing with at that time. They could only be released at the teacher's discretion and it was found that the hyperactive children could be trained very gradually, to play for an increasing length of time if they had the security of the small gate behind them and for short periods they were not given the opportunity to wander aimlessly about the room. Needless to say the table was never used as a punishment and the activities done there were always attractive ones.

The toys on the children's shelves included a wide variety of posting boxes, threading toys, construction toys, matching and grading toys, noisy toys to hit, and stacking and nesting toys. All these would help the children to be aware of size and shape and would also help them to develop nimble fingers.

Along one wall of this 'texture orientated' play room was a gorgeous feely snake. A child could walk the length of the wall dragging his hand along an undulating strip of different feels. One can imagine this being the

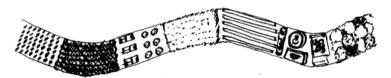

same kind of fun as dragging a stick along a wooden fence, and it is an idea which may appeal to parents and children as a form of decoration on a hall or staircase wall. The snake on the Unit wall consisted of oblongs of these textures:

Woolly balls	assorted pasta shapes
bunches of tissues	cornflakes
sprinkled with perfume	fur
strips of macaroni	sponge
buttons	carpeting
sandpaper	half marbles
polythene packing	shiny card
Scotchbrite scourer	cotton wool balls
stones and shells	foil
dried herbs	rubber
rice	polystyrene

Making Sure Feely Toys are within Reach Blind children are sometimes diffident in reaching out and exploring with their fingers. It may be helpful for

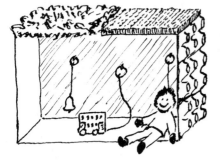

them to play in a confined area such as on a tray with a well defined lip. This prevents the toys from rolling just out of reach. From the blind child's point of view a toy he cannot easily find is as good as gone for ever. In our toy library we make feely boxes and aprons for our very young blind children. The boxes were once grocery cartons but they have been transformed by covering the outside with a variety of feels. E.g. fur fabric, Fablon, bumpy wallpaper, carpet or upholstery samples or sections of egg boxes. Inside are loops of elastic to which can be tied a selection of toys—perhaps whatever is top favourite at the moment, an old friend and something new. The box stands on one of its sides which then becomes its floor. This makes a good surface for building games and bricks cannot topple out of reach but stay confined within the box.

The feely aprons are made from gay nursery fabric with strings to tie round necks and waists so that they will fit all shapes and sizes of child. The bottom is turned up to make a deep pocket (like a Pelican bib) which will hold a collection of treasures. Across the middle, on the wrong side, is stitched a length of strengthening tape. On the right side are sewn large curtain rings at fairly wide intervals along the tape. These are used to attach toys to, and the selection can be as varied as required. These little aprons have been found to be very useful. As well as serving as cover ups they make sure that the child can always reach something to play with. See also Feely Cushion and Humpty Dumpty Page 111.

SOME WAYS OF ENCOURAGING THE SENSE OF TOUCH IN THE HOME

How can this fundamental urge to handle things be used to the best advantage? For many handicapped children an educated sense of touch is a major asset. Its development can be encouraged from a very early age simply by providing baby with a wide variety of safe and attractive feels.

Children who are immobile can only touch what is put

directly within their reach. This fact seems so obvious that it should not really need stating. Unfortunately it is also a fact that some children can lie or sit for many hours, day after day, with literally nothing to do. This puts a big responsibility on all those concerned with the care of such children. Firstly, they must try to imagine what it is like to be so immobile and dependent on others for every diversion, and then they must use their imagination in trying to provide stimulating play material, however unorthodox this may be.

Helping Babies to Feel
Bought cot toys to suspend across the bars on elastic often consist of brightly coloured plastic shapes with a rattle inside. Excellent as these are, a baby's experience can easily be widened by varying the articles suspended. Even such every day objects as a hair roller, a wooden spoon or a plastic egg cup can make splendid playthings. These 'toys' can be changed as often as required, i.e. when baby is not attracted by them — and a wide range of familiar articles of different shapes

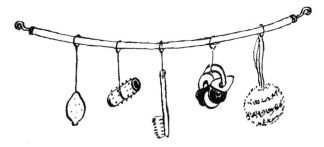

and textures can be offered for his examination. An easy way to suspend cot toys is on a length of bungee rubber with hooks at each end, sold at car accessory or cycle shops for fixing luggage to a carrier. It comes in various lengths so it is wise to measure the cot before buying, and to choose the one which will not need too much tension to keep it taut. The toys can be hung from this by string or by elastic if a bobbing toy is required. For a few children it is safe and sensible to suspend the toy on wire. Pipe cleaners twisted together to make the right length, can be a simple way to achieve this kind of rigid suspension.

With the very young child, because he is not too heavy to lift easily, it is often possible to contrive a normal situation and so give him a chance to learn by experience like his brothers and sisters. Imagine a baby sitting in his pram. His chief amusement is dropping his toys over the side and watching them fall. Soon his Mother ties his toys to the side of the pram so that in theory he can pull them back for himself, but it is still the fun of dropping the toy that pleases him—the relaxing of his grasp and the inevitable drop. He has discovered the eternal truth of the law of gravity and his own power to make things behave in a comfortingly predictable way.

A handicapped child, for a variety of reasons, may never sit up or may be very late in doing so. While he is still physically small and easily handled, he can be given the same chance to enjoy grasping, releasing and dropping with a satisfying clatter. He could perhaps be supported over an adult's shoulder and helped to drop things on to a noisy surface, like an old tin tray. An older brother or sister might willingly act as 'salvage man' to reclaim and return the dropped toys so turning a simple activity into an enjoyable family game.

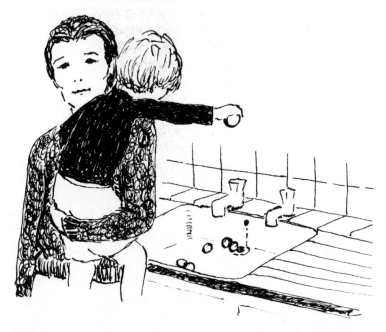

While he is very young a child can be carried about the room and allowed to feel the different surfaces, stroking the soft velvet curtains, bumpy wallpaper, cold kitchen tiles, warm window ledges where the sun has shone, patting the hard wooden table or gripping the smooth round rail at the back of the chair. He may like to be held while he plays with the cold tap. Its shiny surface will attract him and he will enjoy the tickling feel of the gush of water through his fingers.

Helping toddlers to Feel   When he has outgrown the first stages of baby play the toddler is ready to advance to more exciting explorations. If he could express himself sufficiently clearly the average two year old would probably vote for the garbage pail as his favourite toy. Its contents are different every time he gets the chance to explore it and even the fact that it is taboo adds to its attraction. One day there might be a cold shiny pickle jar with an interesting smell, or curly potato peelings or the crackly paper from a box of special biscuits. Another day it

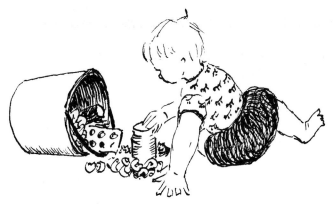

might have an egg box with exciting little pockets in it and a lid to flap about, or bright orange peel or brittle egg shells or a plastic tray from a box of jam tarts. Of course, it is not sensible to use the garbage pail as a toy, but all the things mentioned above might be given to a child to examine and explore before they are considered waste and flung into the bin. By handling such rubbish (under supervision) a child can be realistically involved in daily living and so add to his knowledge of his surroundings. A severely spastic child may never have to peel a potato but he should at least have the chance to know that the mash he enjoys for lunch does not grow that way.

Unwrapping the contents of the shopping basket and if possible, helping to stow the goods away, can be a very useful and informative occupation. Perhaps the shopping can be divided between two bags, one containing breakable items, like eggs and squashable fruit, the other full of tins and packets it is safe to give to a toddler. Through handling the different articles he will learn a lot about size, weight, shape and possibly smell. He will enjoy the fun of taking things out of bags and can learn to recognize articles by the pictures on the wrappers. He may even learn to pick out letters such as his own initial. Meanwhile his hands will have been turning the articles round to help him to examine them and he will be gaining confidence and skill in controlling but not dropping.

Hiding things in Containers. All children love to play with an old handbag and this can be filled with a

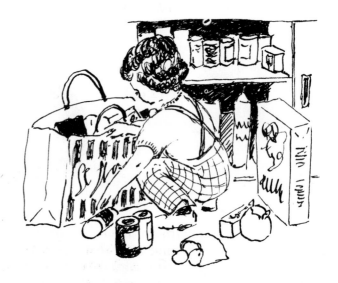

glorious conglomeration of feely articles—perhaps crunchy paper, round shiny conkers, bits of string, large buttons—a real schoolboy's pocket! If feeling and groping inside an old handbag is an absorbing activity which pleases a child, he may like to ring the changes by delving into a carrier bag or an old sock or pillow case to find a treasure. Some children like to wiggle their fingers in a bowl of sand, lentils, sawdust or dried peas and scrabble about to find a hidden toy. Others like to fish in a bowl of soapsuds to find a surprise. This can be a good activity for bath time if bubble bath is used in a small basin. All the inevitable drips and splashes fall harmlessly into the big bath where they can then be put to their proper use!

Making a Special 'Feely' Corner

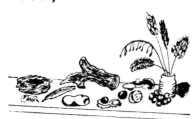

In Nursery and First schools one can often find a Nature Table or an Interest Table or a Destruction Table (where things such as old clocks, can be taken apart without dire consequences). Such tables are set apart for a specific purpose, to focus the childrens' attention in a certain direction. The idea can profitably be copied in many homes where a corner, a small table or window ledge can be reserved for special things and the 'display' changed as necessary. Such areas can become the beginnings of a museum or collectors' corner if the child's interest turns in this direction, but at first it may well be just a fun shelf where the family can enjoy special things worth examining.

As this chapter is discussing touch the articles on the shelf might be a conker with its prickly shell, or a large smooth pebble or a sponge rubber toy or a piece of polystyrene tile broken into a strange shape. Wood, metal, feathers, fur, plastic—all could find a place. Obviously the contents of the shelf will depend on the interests and needs of the child for whom it is designed. To put something new on the shelf while the child is at school can be a way of welcoming him home to a happy surprise.

As a child's hands develop and enlarge he learns to control them with more accuracy. He discovers how to use his finger tips with delicacy and precision. Watch a two year old try to push shapes through the lid of a posting box. Even if he gets the correct shape near the hole the chances are he will try to force it through with the palm of his hand. Soon his four year old brother will be able to stand by watching no longer. This child will pick up the shape with his thumb and finger tips, place it correctly in line with the hole and neatly pop it in.

During these early years a child makes many hundreds of discoveries about the difference between hot and cold, rough and smooth, heavy and light, soft and hard, and nearly all this learning comes through his busy fingers. Later he learns to write—to communicate and record—and he can become proficient in a special skill like playing a musical instrument or model making. Again his nimble fingers are the secret of his success. The more these fingers can be encouraged to develop such fine co-ordinated movements, strength and nimbleness, the more pleasure through creativeness can the child enjoy.

'INSTANT' TOYS AND ACTIVITIES WHICH ENCOURAGE CHILDREN TO USE THEIR FINGERS

The following ideas can be used to fill odd moments or cheer up a dreary day when something new to do can often save a child from boredom and bad temper. All are devised from junk or household items.

FEELY GAMES TO PLAY

Some Variations of Kim's Game

Put an assortment of articles in a container like an old sock or thick stocking or pillowcase. Secure the end and let the child guess what is hidden inside. Open the end and let him rummage inside to see if he is right.

Let the child place some articles on a tray so that he already knows the shape and texture of them. Cover these with a cloth and re-arrange them so that the child cannot remember where they should be. Let him feel through the cloth and find the egg cup or the nailbrush etc. For children who cannot resist peeping, putting the tray of articles inside an old pillowcase will solve this difficulty!

Guess What?

Sit at a table and have a few feely articles on your lap. All hands must be kept under the table. Pass the child an article to examine and identify with his fingers, not looking at it until he has tried to name it—then he can check his guess.

Treasure Hunt

This is a good game to play out of doors. Ask the child to find a particular thing and give him some positive encouragement every time he is successful. (This could be by making a small cairn of stones, adding another stone for each successful mission, or marking ticks in a patch of smooth dry earth, or making a miniature fence of twigs—anything to mark his achievement and show the child it is worth while to search for the next object. If this game is played on a Common treasures to find might be a round stone, a blade of grass as long as an arm, a feather, a fir cone, an acorn or a conker, a yellow flower or a leaf as big as a finger nail. This list includes hard, soft, sturdy, delicate, large and small things and consequently is giving the child practice in handling a variety of feels.

Playing with Clothes Pegs

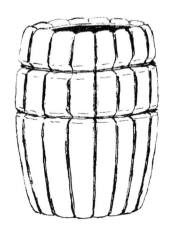

These can be clipped end to end to make a 'monster' or clipped to the lip of an old tin. Ten can be clipped on and then removed one at a time to the tune of 'Ten Green Bottles, hanging on the Wall'. A piece of string can be stretched between two pieces of furniture. Children love to peg up handkerchiefs, bits of rag, dolls clothes, or even pieces of paper to be the washing. Children who are good at paper tearing can tear the shapes of clothes from old newspapers and peg those up. Attractive pots to hold spare pencils etc. can be made from empty baby food tins and split clothes pegs. Wash the tin and make sure there are no sharp edges at the open end. Put two rubber bands (fairly strong ones—or rings of elastic) round the tin. Split a few clothes pegs and poke the halves under the bands until the whole of the outside of the tin is covered with wood. To hold the pieces of wood firmly in place thin copper wire can be twisted round and the sharp ends flattened down and then the elastic bands can be removed. (This is usually a job for a Grownup.) If the wire is not available, button thread or thin string can be wound round and tied securely.

Playing with Scraps of Material

Assuming a rag bag is handy, use it to make a rootling box for materials. A small grocery carton is ideal because the scraps do not become too creased. (If space is short a strong carrier bag will be the next best thing.) Put into the box all the small unwanted pieces of cloth, plus any other textures which are scrap, e.g. an odd fur mitten which has lost its partner, off-cuts of plastic foam, pieces of plastic curtaining, a Scotchbrite scourer, odd scraps of lace and other trimmings, off cuts of carpet square—the wider the variety of textures the better.

Feeling the Textures

Young children like to explore this hotch-potch—perhaps arranging the pieces to cover the table, or in a long line down the hall. Smoothing out the pieces to make them lie flat is a good way of involving both hands and encourages a child to stroke the materials with his finger tips so that he really feels the texture.

Sorting and grading

Some children like to sort the scraps picking out the large pieces or the different colours or finding all the pieces that are the same design or the same texture (e.g. cotton, velvet or wool).

Matching

A quick matching game can be made by cutting a sample from several different textures. Put these in your pocket and give them to a child, one at a time, letting him delve into the box to find the same kind of material as his sample.

MORE THINGS TO DO WITH MATERIAL FOR CHILDREN WHO CAN USE SCISSORS

Making a waver

Cut long strips of any thin material and fix these to a short piece of stick such as a cylindrical brick, half of a washing-up mop handle, or even make a handle from the cardboard from the inside of a toilet roll. Tie the strips of material firmly to the stick and the child can have fun waving the lengths of material about. (This idea has been copied from the paper wavers which give children such delight at carnivals and processions. The material does not rustle like the paper wavers but it is longer lasting.) A short handle is suggested as this makes the waver safer and easier to control but a longer stick is more fun! The provider of the handle must decide on a suitable length.

Instant Dolls Clothes

Families of dolls can be made in a moment if old fashioned dolly clothes pegs are available. (These are the ones made of turned wood with a knob on the top and a slit halfway up the bottom, which slides over the washing line). The knob at the top makes the head and a face and hair can be drawn with felt pens. Clothes can be made by folding a piece of thin material in half and cutting out an oblong of the right size—short for a blouse or shirt, longer for a dress and even longer for a bride or evening wear. Cut a small hole (just big enough for the head of the peg to go through) in the centre of the folded edge. Twist a pipe cleaner round the neck to make arms, open the material out and slip the head

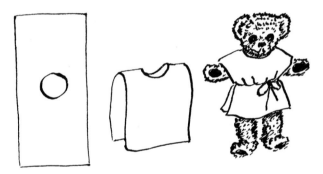

through. Tie the dress down with a belt of wool. Should clothes pegs not be available real dolls or doll shapes cut from cardboard can still be dressed this simple way with no sewing involved. Two bored children discovered this for themselves. One decided to make a uniform for his Action man and spent a happy afternoon devising this. His sister dressed her dolls for a party using dainty scraps of flimsy materials, fraying out the edges to make attractive fringes.

Making Dolls Beds

This is an everpopular game and often leads to playing hospitals or boarding schools. Cardboard boxes to fit the dolls are the first requirement. These can be match boxes, date boxes, shoe boxes, empty soap powder and cereal packets. To make beds for a hospital ward *quantity* is what matters. Paper tissues make ideal sheets and can be folded up for pillows. Oblongs of material can be used for blankets and bed covers and small pieces cut into diet cloths and feeders. The doll patients are certain to have frequent doses of medicine and injections but they might also like some toys. The contents of the rag bag may suggest possibilities but one well tried favourite is making small scrap books using old Christmas cards and empty stamp books to stick the pictures in.

Collage Pictures

Fuzzy Felt games are popular with many children, but some find the pieces too small to handle conveniently, For them, shapes cut from the Rag Rootling Box may be more satisfactory as well as giving them experience with different textures. Left to his own devices a child may aimlessly snip up scraps of material without any real idea of making a picture and he may need some help in getting started. Providing a suitable background can often do the trick. Peter was given a piece from the leg of an old pair of dark grey school trousers. This reminded him of the sky at night and as the month happened to be November his fabric picture included a bonfire and spots of bright materials to represent fireworks, Angela started off with a piece of hessian. This made her think of soil so her picture was of a garden full of fabric flowers with green wool stalks. Simple ideas for beginners might be:-

(a) Making an all over pattern like a patchwork, covering all the background with scraps of material.

(b) Using the background as part of the picture to make e.g. a face —
Cut two ovals for eyes
Cut two halfmoon shapes for eyebrows
A triangle for the nose
A half moon for a smiley mouth
Lengths of wool round the edge for hair.
Or for a house;
Cut a large oblong for the door
Cut a smaller oblongs or squares for windows
Cut thin strips for curtains if required.
Add a chimney,

a crazy paving path,
an herbacious border etc.
(c) Making a design using contrasting textures such as foam rubber and needlecord.

Hints

Do not let the child be in too much of a hurry to stick his picture down. By moving the pieces about a little he may find an arrangement he likes better, and once glue has been used it is difficult to change the design without it looking too messy.

Use School Glue which is available at most stationers. This is water soluble and will wash off clothes. Copydex, which is an excellent fabric adhesive, requires a special solvent so is not suitable for messy workers. Children who are not over fussy about the finished look of their fabric pictures may find ordinary Polycel wallpaper paste quite suitable. It is much cheaper, can be mixed up when required, and is easy to apply. The disadvantages are that it makes the materials wet, can cause colours to run, and alters the appearance of the picture if delicate textures like velvet or thin nylon are used.

Feely Pictures for an Adult to Make

A teacher at a residential school for the blind makes many such pictures for the childrens' bedrooms. She uses as many textures and stimulating feels as she can think of. Using large sheets of cardboard for backing she makes designs with natural materials such as leaves or seaweed, fircones and seeds, and creates pictures such as 'The Hay Cart'. Here the cart is made from twigs, the wheels from the lid of a margarine tub with drinking straws for the spokes. The driver and horse are made from bound rope with strips of leather for the harness and material for the driver's clothes. The cart is filled with real hay. Another feely picture might be of a tree made from real twigs with birds, butterflies, leaves or flowers attached. Decorative birds, butterflies and insects, dried grasses etc can be bought at many florists.

THREADING

Threading is an excellent activity for encouraging fine

93

finger control. The threader must be accurately aimed at the hole which has to be held steady and the threader must be grasped with the finger tips before it is pulled through. Success is measured by the number of articles on the threader and many children enjoy the challenge of making this as long as possible.

Threading Anything

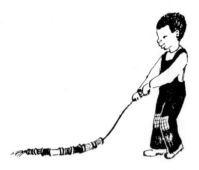

Toddlers at the stage of enjoying towing a toy behind them like to thread up a 'clanky'. This is a collection of objects—noisy ones usually being the most popular—which are threaded onto a piece of stout string and then dragged vigorously up and down the garden path. Any scrap object might be suitable to thread—perhaps an old saucepan lid, an odd sandal or a cardboard cylinder—as long as it has a hole in it and is genuine scrap it is suitable for a 'clanky'. Threading thick string through a large hole can be quite difficult for small fingers but the effort is worth it when the creation can be dragged triumphantly at top speed, giving the child an exhilarating sense of power. See also page 72.

A Cotton Reel Snake

Threading cotton reels on a piece of string (or better still, on a length of plastic earth wire sleeving sold at electrical shops) to make a long snake to pull along makes a good toy for a lively three year old or for an older child to make for his toddler brother. If the child finds the weight of the reels already on the thread tends to pull the thread out of the reel he is trying to add, let him try working at a table. The threaded reels can be supported and he can lie each new reel on its side and poke the threads through—like a train going through a tunnel. Scraps of fablon stuck round the cotton reels make them more attractive and children love peeling off the paper backing before sticking them on. The reels can also be painted gay colours using Humbrol enamel which is non-poisonous.

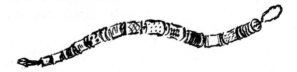

Threading Buttons

Children who can safely handle a pointed needle enjoy this. Buttons can be threaded to make a long string or they can be sorted for colour (an egg box is excellent for this job) and then threaded in order.

Threading on a Pipe cleaner Cut a few plastic drinking straws into short lengths and put them in a saucer so that they are easier to pick up and do not roll all over the table. Nimble fingered children like to thread these tiny pieces onto a pipe cleaner to make a bracelet for themselves or their dolls.

Once a child has sufficient dexterity to thread efficiently he can try activities more like sewing which involves poking a thread in and *out,* which is more difficult than threading.

PRE-SEWING ACTIVITIES

Threading on Peg Board An off cut of peg board (about a foot square) and a length of brightly coloured plastic-covered electrician's wire will give a good introduction to sewing. Tie a bead or cotton reel to the end of the wire so that it cannot pull right through and it can then be threaded in and out of the holes until it is quite used up.

Sewing Cards These can be bought at many toy shops, but it is easy to make very simple ones and these are often better for beginners and slow learners. Use a piece of cardboard, if possible plain on both sides, such as shirt stiffener, the back of a writing pad or a very simple outline shape, larger is available. Draw a very simple outline shape, perhaps a kite or boat or Christmas tree, or just a geometric shape. Decide where the holes for the stitches must go (at all corners and evenly spaced in between) and mark them in pencil. Put the card on a soft surface, such as a thick piled carpet, and poke holes for the stitches with a skewer or a thin knitting needle. Turn the card over and draw the picture again on the back using the holes as guides. The child will find this second picture very helpful when he has to poke the thread back to the front of the card. A blunt needle and wool used double (or with the needle tied on) is suitable for the sewing and as the child becomes proficient he can use several different colours to make the finished picture more attractive. Neatly sewn cards can be used to hang calendars from and given to admiring relatives and friends.

Christmas Card Bags

Choose a pretty card and punch holes through both the front and back of the card about $\frac{1}{2}$" in from the sides and bottom. The child can either sew the card into a little bag using the 'in-out' of running stitch or by going over and over. If he leaves a 'tail' at the beginning and end of his sewing these ends can be tied together to make a handle for the bag.

SEWING ON MATERIAL

Rug Canvas

Because of its large squares some children find this easiest to manage. Double quick knit wool and a curved raffia needle with a blunt end make rows of running stitch fairly easy to do and the finished work can be made into a mat, bag, purse, needlebook, comb case, etc. (Note: fine canvas, such as tapestry canvas, is not suitable for young children to use as it is too dazzling and difficult to aim for the holes.)

Binka Canvas

This is ideal for first real sewing. The holes ensure even stitches and it can be bought in pretty colours from many craft and needlework shops. Use a blunt tapestry needle and preferably *twisted* embroidery cotton (not stranded which tends to separate) or fairly thick wool.
   Older children proficient at cross stitch like to try out their own designs first on peg board as described above.

USING THE SENSE OF TOUCH TO MAKE PATTERNS PICTURES AND MODELS

Salt Drawings

(*WARNING:* Do not try this if the child's hands have any cuts or sore places, as the salt will make these smart.)
Salt drawing makes an excellent introduction to finger

painting and while it is not so exciting or permanent as that it encourages the same large finger movements and is definitely less messy! It has advantages over drawing on a tray sprinkled with flour, an activity which is sometimes suggested for severely handicapped children. Salt, being less fine, tends to stay on the tray more successfully and does not fly up into hair, eyes, etc. All you need is a dark coloured tray and a cannister of salt. A small funnel is also a good idea and can be made by cutting the base from a plastic bottle, upending it and using the spout for the neck of the funnel. At clearing up time this can be used to return the salt to the cannister ready for more play another day. If the cannister is too heavy for the child to hold he can dribble the salt over the tray through the funnel. Once the tray is covered he can draw shapes and patterns in the salt with his finger, revealing the dark base of the tray, smooth it over with a ruler or the palm of his hand and start again. He can also draw with a lolly stick, an old paint brush or anything else you can devise.

Flour Paste Finger Painting

The finger movements encouraged by this activity are similar to those used in salt drawing, but it has a different and more fluid feel and the 'creations' can be kept for a short time.

Start with a shiny, brightly coloured background such as an opened out plastic carrier bag with a psychedelic design on it or a large piece of gaudy paper, protected by polythene film. Spread a mixture of flour and water (uncooked) the consistency of thick cream, over the plastic background. This can then be worked about to reveal the coloured background and when the pattern made is sufficiently swirly and satisfying it can be left flat to dry out. It will last for a few days if kept horizontal and undisturbed and then the white parts can be brushed off and the background used again.

Finger Painting

This is a messy occupation best indulged in just before bath time! It is so much enjoyed by young children and the not so able that it is well worth taking the trouble to provide it now and then. First cover the child with a large overall (an old shirt worn back to front can be ideal for a large child) or remove as much clothing as possible if the weather is warm. Make a fairly stiff mixture of flour and water paste or cornflour paste and divide the mixture into two containers (yogurt pots are excellent). Add a different coloured powder paint to each pot—e.g. blue and yellow. Put two blobs of paint in the middle of an old tray or on a formica topped table or

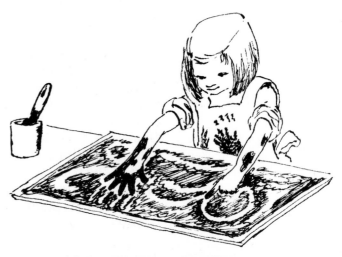

even on an old tin meat plate. The larger the surface the better. The child can swirl the paint about, mixing the colours together and drag his fingers through the sticky film to show clear areas of table top. The paint can be squeezed up into little walls and then squashed and smeared flat again, giving a chance to experiment in colour blending. See Basic Recipes Page 147 for more detailed ways of making finger paint.

Making a Snail Trail

Fill a polythene bag with finger paint, tie up the top, snip the corner off and let the child squeeze the bag to force the paint in a squiggly line over a large sheet of paper—rather like squirting icing out of a forcing bag.

Making a Collage
(*See also P. 92*)

Making a picture or pattern using an assortment of different materials of varying textures is an excellent way of letting a child use these imaginatively. A feely collage can be very simple—perhaps filling half of an old cheese box with play pastry or Polyfilla and poking in things like buttons or butter beans or pieces of match stick to make a design.

Another simple texture pattern can be made by soaking some fairly thick string or wool in Polycell paste or Gloy and then arranging it on a piece of cardboard to make interesting spaces. The string should be left to dry and stick firmly to the cardboard and then the spaces can be filled in with different textures—perhaps torn pieces of bubbly wallpaper or seeds—one area could be covered with rice, another with lentils, another with split peas or butter beans. Various shapes of Pasta can make excellent collages too.

Cutting out a large paper doll from thin card and letting a child dress it by sticking on pieces of material of different kinds can help him to appreciate the difference between various fabrics—as well as helping his vocabulary of words for parts of the body and the appropriate clothes.

Simple collage pictures are easy to make once the knack has been developed, and can look very spectacular even if the technique of the artist is not very developed. Imagine cheering up a dull February day by making a collage of a window box. The background might be the cardboard from the side of a grocery carton. (If there is printing on it this can be covered by making powder paint the consistency of double cream, by using a mixture of half washing-up liquid and half water to add to the paint.) The window box might be made from the side of a cornflakes box. The flowers could be painted sections from an egg box with shiny milk bottle top centres, the stalks could be drinking straws or pipe cleaners and the leaves cut from stiff paper or material. Two dimensional flowers can be cut from old Christmas cards or Seedsmen's catalogues.

Fabric collages can be stuck with School Glue (water solvent), or Copydex, or sewn, according to the child's skill and the nature of the design.

MODELLING

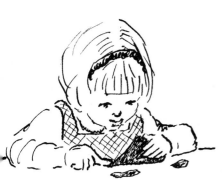

This activity makes use of both hands in a way which most children find very satisfying.

Severely handicapped children often discover that modelling (working in three dimensions) is easier for them than drawing or painting and with experience they can achieve very pleasing results. At first they may only squeeze, slap, poke or break the modelling material into tiny pieces but gradually they will discover for themselves more exciting ways of using it and can be shown other things to do. Some parents may feel disinclined to provide modelling materials for their children. Perhaps when they were young they missed the opportunity of this sort of creativity and may worry that they may not be able to help their child, or perhaps they dread a mess. It is just this element of messiness which makes modelling so popular with many children, who cannot get grubby through their normal play. Not for them are the toddlers' joy in exploring the coal bucket, stamping in puddles or dragging a stick through the mud; they will miss out on the later pleasures of cooking and messing about with oily bicycles, but playing with a satisfyingly large lump of clay or play pastry may be some slight compensation and may lead to real skill and fulfilment in these media.

Sand

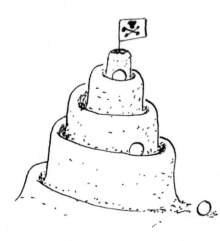

Sand casting

Used damp so that it will not fly up into eyes and noses, this makes a perfect substance for early play. It has no form of its own so a child can mould it as he wishes—at first just filling up containers or smoothing it down, endlessly piling it up and flattening it. Most children soon discover more exciting ways of using it.

Storing it can be a problem but parents with a garden have found that an old motor tyre makes a good rim for a sand pit. This can be scrubbed and painted and is easy to cover over with a sheet of plastic to keep the rain (and cats) away. A school for SSN children uses a tractor tyre, painted white, as a sand pit.

Damp sand is perfect for first attempts at modelling—perhaps just making roadways with 'hedges' for model cars or piling the sand up into little mounds. Older children may use these same skills in a more advanced way, modelling raised faces like masks or making a ball race round the outside of a large castle.

If sand is not available, damp sawdust makes a splendid substitute and can be moulded just like sand.

Damp sand can also be used for making simple casts—perhaps of a hand print, or a footprint, or any other interesting shape like the prickly case of a horse-chestnut conker, or the pattern on the sole of a gum boot. Prepare a very flat patch of damp sand and clear away all tiny stones. Build a low wall of sand round the area where the cast will be made. For a hand print press the hand gently but firmly into the damp sand, making a distinct depression. Adjust the position of the wall to make a frame to fit round the hand print and gently pour in some plaster of Paris (bought in 7lb bags from an ironmonger) or Polyfilla (more expensive for a much smaller quantity). The amount of plaster used will depend on the size of the shape cast. It must not be too thin or it will snap. Leave the plaster to set. This will take at least 15–30 minutes. It is easier to handle if left for considerably longer until it has really set hard, but children are usually impatient to see the result and with care it can be gently raised while still damp. It looks slightly off white until it is quite dry. The hand print on the plaster will be a raised one. When it is quite dry any sand left sticking to it can be gently brushed away. Wall plaques can be made by this same method and painted. A small loop of bent wire for hanging each plaque can be embedded in the plaster before it sets. Patterned plaques can be made by pressing shapes in the firm damp sand. The edge of a ruler, a cotton reel, a split clothes peg—these are just a few shapes which work successfully.

Play Pastry

This is excellent as an introduction to more sophisticated modelling materials. It is easy to make at any time when it is needed and is splendid for poking, pinching, squeezing and making into simple shapes, such as potatoes or carrots for a shop, or play sweets to wrap in pretty papers to use with a weighing machine. It will dry quite hard and can be painted, but as with ordinary clay, thin shapes will be brittle. It is quite harmless (but not very appetizing should the modeller be tempted to eat some). When dry it sometimes tends to crack so if a child insists on moulding a long thin worm, let him use a pipe cleaner as a backbone to model it round and he is less likely to be disappointed in the finished article. Play pastry can be used very satisfactorily in conjunction with other materials. e.g. A feely hedgehog is simple to make. A child can model the shape of a hedgehog with the pastry using a piece of cardboard as a base board. (This makes it easier to handle the finished model.) The hedgehog's prickles can be made with needles from a Pine tree or with drinking straws or match sticks or cocktail sticks (with the sharp tips removed), his eyes can be made from seeds from a fir cone, currants or even dabs of paint. When he is finished he can have pride of place in the 'feely corner'. See page 87.

Recipe for Play Pastry

Two cups of flour
About $\frac{1}{2}$ cup of salt (this helps to keep the flour fresh)
2 teaspoons cooking oil (optional but it makes a better texture)
Enough water to mix to the consistency of ordinary pastry

Play pastry must not be sticky. It should leave the fingers quite clean when it is handled. It is fun to make coloured pastry sometimes. Half the flour and salt can be mixed with plain water and half with coloured water. Use powder paint or cooking colouring—e.g. cochineal. Play pastry can be used many times over if it is stored in a plastic bag in the fridge.

Mud and Clay

These make splendid modelling materials. If used at the right texture, not too dry and crumbly and not too 'sloppy', clay need not be very messy. It is one of the best substances for modelling because it can give satisfactory results whatever the skill of its user. It takes less patience than papier mâché or Plasticine which can be stiff to handle in large quantities. Clay, packed in a neat polythene bucket with a lid, complete with tools, hardener and suggestions for use, can be bought from large toy and craft shops. The Fulham Pottery Ltd, Dept C2, 210 New Kings Road, London SW6 4NY supply 'cold clay' which dries very hard like fired clay. If it is left to dry out it can be made useable again just by adding water.

Plasticine

A new packet of this well-loved material with its

distinctive smell and the bright coloured strips of very manageable modelling substance is popular with many children with particularly nimble fingers. (See Rachel Page 3.) It is expensive to provide in sizable quantities. For some children it can be too stiff, particularly when it is ageing or the weather is cold. The lovely colours tend to merge with use but older children who want to make models to keep will find it entirely satisfactory.

Papier Mâché

It is possible to make a useful paper pulp which can be used like clay but is much lighter when it has dried out. This makes it very suitable for glove puppet heads. It has one great drawback in that it is very tedious to make and takes a long time. For children who want quick results it is useless, but for children who enjoy tearing up the required volume of paper it can be very successful.

Tear newspaper (not pages from magazines which are shiny) into small pieces about the size of a postage stamp. The paper must not be cut, but torn as this gives a jagged edge which helps to break down the fibres. Put the scraps of paper in a galvanized bucket and cover with cold water. Leave it to soak for about three weeks and then bring it to the boil and simmer it for at least two hours. Make sure the water does not boil away and occasionally stir the mixture carefully with a stick, leave it to cool and drain off all the surplus water. When you want to use this mixture for modelling add flour paste, and if possible, whitening. This is powdered chalk and is obtainable from some builders' merchants. It improves the colour of the paper pulp and adds to its bulk. To pulp made from a bucket full of torn paper add 1lb whitening and the following amount of flour paste:-

Use 1 cupful of plain flour
1 oz Alum (from a chemist)
Mix these to a smooth paste with cold water
Add 1 pint of cold water

Bring slowly to the boil, stirring all the time to prevent lumps. The mixture will gradually thicken. Boil it gently for about five minutes to cook it thoroughly. When it has cooled it can be stirred well into the paper pulp making sure there are no lumps, and modelling can begin. This is the way to make the best papier mâché, which should be really smooth and free from lumps. If all you need is a cheap squelchy modelling material you can cut down on the soaking time and even leave out the boiling up.

Another way of using paper for modelling by sticking it on in layers is described on page 69, Homemade Noisemakers. Children enjoy making small pots and dishes by this method and providing they are reasonably patient and take care to smooth out the strips of paper and there are no ugly ridges they can achieve very good results.

You will need a mould to model over—a saucer will make a dish, a jam jar covered about ⅔rds of the way up its sides will make a plant holder or a pot to keep felt pens in. Avoid a shape with a turned in tip or the finished papier mâché shape cannot be taken off the mould. You will also need a supply of newspaper and soft paper like tissue paper (bread wrapping will do), vaseline or flour paste.

Turn the mould upside down if the outside is going to be used to form the shape e.g. with a jam jar. With a saucer either side could be used, but an inverted saucer is more stable for working on. Smear the mould with vaseline to stop the first layer of paper from sticking to it. Tear the paper into small pieces; do not bother to paste these but let them stick on the mould with the vaseline. Cover this layer with another pasted layer of scraps of paper making sure it is evenly covered all over, otherwise the finished article will have thin places and may crack. It is helpful to use alternate layers of newspaper and some other unglazed paper, so that it is easy to tell when each layer is properly finished. Eight layers of paper will make a fairly sturdy article. Large shapes need more layers. Finishing off with layers of tissue paper gives a smoother surface which is better for painting. When it has quite dried out, take the model off the mould. Trim the lip with scissors and stick more paper over the inside greasy surface to neaten it and make it paintable. When the model is quite dry it can be decorated. If the final layer of paper has been white this can be painted straight away but if the newspaper still shows it is worthwhile covering this up with a coat of emulsion paint. When this is dry poster or powder paints can be used for the decoration. Some coats of Polyurethane varnish will protect the model and make it spongeable. Sufficient layers of varnish should make it waterproof.

HELPING A CHILD TO USE A 'LAZY HAND'

It is very difficult to make sensible suggestions for an unknown child, but the following toys and activities all need the use of both hands and may be suitable for some children who have a 'lazy' hand, capable of movement, but because it is less efficient than the 'good' hand it tends to be ignored. While this is primarily a problem for discussion with the child's therapist there are many play ways through which the use of both hands can be encouraged. Perhaps your child is like Sarah, a three year old whose left arm and hand were quite useable but because she could manage her right hand so much more efficiently she tended to 'carry' her left one, holding it close to her body with the elbow bent. This became a habit which her therapist explained it was important to break as soon as possible. The first toy to be successful with her was a set of large light building bricks. These were made from empty soap boxes collected from all the neighbours, and before the tops were taped down they were stuffed with crunched up newspaper to make them stronger. With these large bricks Sarah was able to build a stack, make steps, arrange them to make chairs for her dolls or build them into shelters for her farm animals. Because of the size of each brick it was impossible for her to use only one hand, and the 'lazy' one had to be used as a pusher. This led on to building with large empty cartons which could be piled up or nested inside each other and finally jumped on! Pushing a pram was a failure with Sarah because she could manage fairly well with only one hand but wheeling a barrow or steering a tricycle was only possible when she could use both.

The following 'two handed' activities have all worked with many children and may provide you with some fresh ideas.

PLAY HELPS

About the House

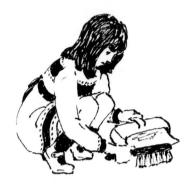

Think of all the jobs you can only do using both hands and help your child to imitate you in such tasks as

(a) shaking and folding a manageable piece of material like a serviette or a tray cloth. Folding handkerchiefs or the baby's nappies.

(b) hanging up the washing. The real washing line will be too high for most children, but a play line can be strung between two convenient points and the child can peg out small light items like his own socks and handkerchiefs. 'Washing Day' makes a good game for indoors too. A string line can be stretched between the backs of two chairs and pretend washing hung up. See page 89.

(c) using a rolling pin, preferably a real one with handles at each end. This is sufficiently heavy to make an impression on the dough leaving the child free to concentrate on rolling straight. For the recipe for play pastry see page 148.

(d) carrying an empty tray, progressing to managing a tray with something unbreakable on it, finally being skilful enough to carry liquid on a tray.

(e) using a dustpan and brush.

(f) taking the lids off screw top jars.

At Bath Time

(a) put a floating toy in the bath and let the child make it 'swim' round him as he swishes the water, pulling with one hand and pushing with the other. He can change the direction in which the toy travels by reversing the movement of his hands and arms.

(b) put a small plastic bowl to float on the surface of the water and let the child use this like a steering wheel. Watch out for floor flooding!

(c) cut a washing up detergent bottle in half. The top turned upside down will make a funnel and the bottom can be used to fill this up. Children love to direct the flow of water to trickle onto their knees and toes. Pouring water through a sieve or colander is also very popular. The water seems to disappear like magic.

Other Toys and Activities to Encourage the Use of Both Hands

(a) a hoop. This can be used as a tool to hook things nearer, or it can be used to push a large ball along. Passing it over the head and shoulders can also be a good exercise but this is not really much *fun.* Putting on

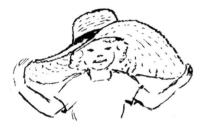

a large glamourous wide-brimmed hat may well have more child appeal!

(b) playing with a large plastic inflated beach ball is a well-tried winner.

(c) threading things. Some children are not attracted to the usual bead threading and lacing activities. They may prefer to thread a Clanky see page 72, or even threading a collection of keys on some thick string. A rigid tag which will last long enough for poking through the key handles can be made by winding Sellotape tightly round the end of the string.

(d) Some children are happy to thread a plastic tube (made from a detergent bottle with the top and bottom cut off) over their 'lazy' hand and if a face is drawn on this first a game of 'Peep-bo' with the hand popping out of the top of the tube can make a happy diversion.

(e) Puppets are worth trying too. A child will often hold his hand up and wave it about if it is disguised as something else. Glove puppets are quite hard to manipulate, but paper bag puppets or sock puppets can be very successful. (See pages 31 and 33.)

(f) Construction sets must be large and simple. Nuts and bolts can be discouraging, but large shapes to poke together to make a spectacular result may well be successful. The ESA Wooden Construction Set or 'Matador' (from some large toy shops and by mail order) are big and chunky for beginners and could lead on to other construction sets such as Tinker Toy which has smaller solid shapes and thinner connecting rods. 'Construct-O-Straws' are less robust, but are very light and easy to handle and can be fun for older children. They are popular with a Toy Library member who has brittle bones, and with another who has muscular dystrophy.

(g) All cutting out activities involving the use of scissors can be helpful. For children who cannot manage ordinary scissors ESA market a special pair with a spring for a handle. It is in their catalogue of 'Play Extra Specials.'

(h) All filing activities such as sculpting a block of balsa wood, rock salt, chalk or Plaster of Paris.

(i) Playing some musical instruments like a *pair* of maraccas, hitting a triangle, or clashing the cymbals.

(j) Many forms of physical activity can be successful, from clapping hands in a game of pat-a-cake to more strenuous skipping, swimming, climbing, archery, riding or rowing a rubber inflatable dinghy tethered by a rope.

There are a few other bought toys which can only be manipulated with both hands. E.g. Galts climbing man rises up two lengths of string when they are pulled alternately, and there are other old favourites like stencils to colour in, Etch-a-sketch with its two knobs to twiddle, and Rotadraw where the plastic disc must be controlled by one hand while the other fills in the lines. Mr Potato Head is worth trying too. This is a very cheap toy with a limited span of life, but it can give great pleasure. Plastic features on spikes must be poked into a potato to make a funny face. If a child is not strong enough to push into a potato a ball of play pastry (see page 148) will do just as well. The potato—or pastry—can be held in the 'lazy' hand.

Worth mentioning too are all the craft activities like sewing, knitting, weaving, and basketry. For children who find these too hard Origami paper folding might be possible.

PLAY FOR CHILDREN WHO CAN USE ONLY ONE HAND

The ideas in this section are suggested for children who have injured one hand, or who have never had the use of two. Making their playtime more exciting may often be just a question of organization and adaption. E.g. Mixing and stirring in a basin is possible if the bowl rests on a Dycem non-slip mat (available from some large stores, ESA and the Spastics' Society, 12 Park Crescent, London WIN 4EQ). Older children can carve or file soap or balsa if these are supported on a long nail stuck through a stable base board and Four to Eight have thought of the clever idea of putting a drawing pin on some pieces of wooden puzzle so that these can be manipulated with a magnet.

(a) All throwing games are usually possible. Large plastic skittles to knock down with a bean bag (easier to hold for some children) may be just right for a young child; one a little more skilful may prefer a game of marbles while a teenager might be more interested in playing darts. There are many more similar aiming games of varying difficulty such as Quoits for the active or Ring Toss for the less mobile. Children can become very skilled at these games and they can be an excellent way of encouraging play with other children.

(b) All building games have possibilities for one handed children. The traditional wooden building bricks are fairly heavy and stable and can be used in conjunction with model cars or farm animals for 'let's pretend' games. Plastic bricks are lighter and more suitable for some children and large sponge rubber bricks (for non-biters) can be bought or made from off cuts, and the child can pinch into these to get a firm grip. Sticklebricks can be pressed together to make shapes, but can be hard to take apart again. Most children use their teeth to help! Interlocking bricks like Lego are excellent for more able children who can build exciting structures on the base boards provided. Lego can be bought in different sizes of brick which can all be used together, so the set can be added to as the need arises. Galts produce a magnetic building set which older children find fascinating.

(c) All peg games can be managed with one hand. These vary from peg boards of different sizes, with 50 or 100 holes, where coloured pegs can be arranged in patterns, to games of skill for older children like Mastermind. Full sized Chess and Draughts sets with pegs on each piece and holes in the board can be obtained from The Royal National Institute for the Blind, 224-8 Great Portland Street London W1. Several other toys also have pegs on parts which fit into holes. One is a large jigsaw of a seaside and there are houses, trees, boats etc to fit into the jigsaw base. This is made by Kiddicraft and available at some shops. Down on the Farm is sold by Thomas Hope Ltd Royton Ring Mill, St Phillips Drive, Royton, Oldham, Lancashire, and consists of a generous supply of animals and people which peg into green plastic bases.

(d) All magnetic games can be controlled with one hand. These can be bought at many toy shops or through several of the suppliers listed on page 165. The Toy Libraries Association publishes a leaflet called 'Magnetic Toys' which includes information on how to make your own and where to buy different sorts of magnets and metal boards. When buying a magnetic game in a shop select one with magnets that are powerful enough to stick firmly to the board. Velcro (sold at haberdashery departments and often used on callipers etc) can sometimes serve the same purpose as a magnet and is much cheaper. It is excellent if firmly sewn to material, but tends to pull away from wood or cardboard.

(e) All sliding games where the pieces need manoeuvring into position, such as pattern making with mosaic shapes. Non-interlocking jig-saws can be fun if a tray with a beading round it is used as a play surface. The pieces can be slid into position against the edging.

(f) All dice games from simple ones like Rainbow Towers which only involves colour matching, to complicated ones like Monopoly can all be played with one hand.

(g) Card games are possible if the child can have a card holder. This can be made by putting several deep saw cuts parallel to each other at an angle across a solid piece of wood or one can be bought from the Red Cross. In an emergency cards can be planted in the upturned bristles of a scrubbing brush.

As you dip into other parts of this book you will find many suggestions which may be just right for your child. Perhaps he would enjoy poking shapes into play pastry, or printing, or shaking a rattle in time to music on the radio. If the weather is warm and he is wearing the minimum of play clothes he might like to 'paint' the coal bunker with an old distemper brush and a bucket of water or let off steam by running around towing a Clanky.

**Bought Toys
Specially Suitable for
the One Handed**

All hammer toys—particularly the Ball Hammer Toy where four little wooden balls rest on holes with soft plastic washers round the edge. When the balls are banged they disappear inside the toy and roll out at a small hole at the side.

All Pile Ups—King of the Castle is a specially good one because the shapes have a ridge at the top which makes the tower very stable and is useful for picking up the pieces.

Squeeze Toys from Fisher Price. A large plastic bulb must be pressed to make the frog hop etc.

Marbles and Marble Games such as Solitaire and Builda Helta Skelta.

Bagatelle for those old enough to enjoy scoring games.

A Yo Yo makes a good stocking filler!

A Rolf Harris Stylophone obtainable from music shops and large toy shops is an expensive toy but can give great pleasure to children who like to pick out tunes. The tiny notes will play when they are touched with the stylus. The Stylophone is battery operated so requires very little effort to produce the sound which makes it a good instrument for children who have not the strength to blow a recorder or play a guitar etc.

HOMEMADE TOYS FOR TOUCH

Feely Cushion

This can make a good toy for a baby providing it is *firmly tied on to the cot bars and there can be no danger of the child pulling it over his face.* If you are not fond of sewing use a scatter cushion, foam filled, with a detatchable cover which is washable. Attach a rattle, or a soft toy, or a shiny tea spoon to it by a short length of tape. Ring the changes by offering an old favourite and sometimes something new. If baby is not yet very strong these can be fixed on with short lengths of tape (which must not be long enough to become tangled between tiny fingers) and nappy pins with their special non-prick safety heads. Remember to tie the cushion at least twice at the back of the cot bars, or if the child is playing on the floor it can be securely tied to the leg of a piece of furniture. Play cushions like these are recommended in 'Play in Hospital' by Susan Harvey and Ann Hales-Tooke for babies who are in oxygen tents and easily lose their toys among the bed clothes. They are also very useful for all children who tend to

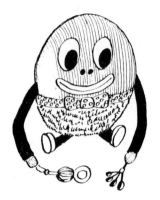

push their toys away and then cannot reach them. If you enjoy sewing and feel in a creative mood you can design a special comfort cushion. This might be in the shape of a Humpty Dumpty who could be firmly fixed in a convenient position, and every day he could hold in his hands a different 'feel' —perhaps a teething ring, or a bunch of plastic measuring spoons, or a wooden spoon. His body might be made of smooth shiny material, his trousers of rough tweed or fur fabric, his legs and arms of ridgy corduroy and his shoes of leather from an old belt. Remember to finish off all ends very securely and to make a good job of the seams. Children love to 'pick' and can work astonishingly fast!

The following group of toys were all made specially for a little girl of six who had recently lost her sight as the result of a brain tumour. The challenge was to devise toys which would help her to use her fingers where formally she had used her eyes, and to help her to be aware of textures through her finger tips. This increased sensitivity would be needed when she was ready to receive education at a school for the blind and learn Braille. Although designed for a blind child, these toys have also given pleasure to many other children, 'normal' and handicapped.

Feely Caterpillar

This was made from circles of materials of different textures and these were joined together in pairs and stuffed with old nylon stockings to make a long line of little round cushions. These were fixed together with squares of Velcro (obtainable from haberdashery departments) and the back half of one segment was made to correspond with the front half of the next so that velvet would join on to velvet, plastic to plastic, needlecord to needlecord etc. Other materials used were fluffy blanket, cotton, a knobbly tweed, silk and terry towelling. It is best to back a piece of thin material with something stronger to prevent the Velcro from tearing it. The front of the caterpillar was indicated with a face made with button eyes and a curtain ring mouth, and the last segment finished off with a tassel tail.

Feely Bingo

This game is played like ordinary Bingo and small cards

are matched to a master card. Instead of pictures or numbers being used, all the cards have different textures. The game is easy to make once all the materials have been gathered together. Start off with a box or tin about 8″ X 10″; (an empty chocolate box or a stocking box from a drapers does very well). This avoids the problem of creating a splendid game with lots of pieces, and then being unable to find anything to keep it in! Cut an even number of pieces of cardboard from a grocery carton, Cornflakes box etc making them as large as possible, but able to fit in the box. If three people are likely to play the game you will need six cards. Raid your rag bag for scraps and keep a lookout for off cuts of different textures from materials used around the house. You might have scraps of the materials mentioned for the Feely Caterpillar, and to these you can add 'feels' like sandpaper, off cuts of carpet, lino tiles, foam rubber and even flat woven pan scrubber. Take a card and firmly stick on squares of four contrasting textures such as sand paper, velvet, fur fabric and lino tile. Repeat these textures on another card and cut this one into four pieces so that the texture

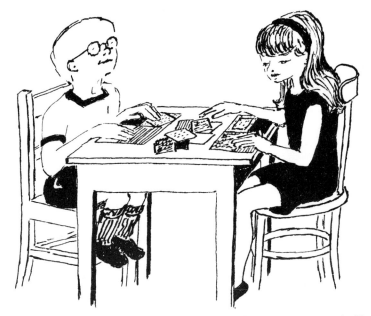

on each piece can be matched to the master card. Do this again with the next pair of cards, using different textures, and make as many pairs of cards as you can with the number of 'feels' available. If this makes the game too complicated for a slow learner some cards can be put by and added to the game gradually.

Feely Dominoes

This game is played like ordinary dominoes, but textures must be matched instead of spots. Cut plenty of oblongs in thick cardboard and stick a 'feel' on each end using any of those mentioned above. You can do this in a haphazard way, or you can copy the real game of dominoes and have one texture to represent each number and arrange the feely dominoes to correspond with conventional ones which go 6,6; 6,5; 6,4; 6,3 etc, then 5,5; 5,4; 5,3, continuing like this until double blank is reached.

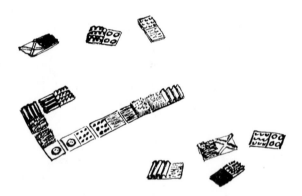

Feely Bags

These make a good doodle toy and as well as being helpful to blind children who like to try to identify the contents, they are also enjoyed by slow learners, and can encourage finger movements by children whose hands are stiff and clumsy. They can be made super strong for 'biters' (by using particularly tough material like deck chair canvas or upholstery material and sewing them with button thread) or filled with light contents for 'throwers'. They are made like bean bags but the material used is chosen for its feely appeal. Ideally it must also be fairly thin so that the contents of the bag are easily felt through the fabric. The idea is to put at least two different fillings in each bag so that the child can separate these by wiggling them about inside the bag. The following fillings have been used for the blind child already mentioned, but some could be very dangerous if given to a destructive child likely to rip open the bags and eat the contents. For such a one edible contents like rice, peas and macaroni would be safer. Some suggested fillings are—

    a slightly inflated balloon
    rice and a few buttons
    two curtain rings and some dried peas
    lentils, orange pips and a marble
    a cotton reel, some coins and a piece of sponge rubber
    spaghetti which can be broken up inside the bag.

Open Sesame Board

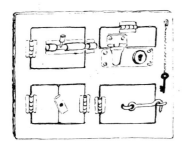

This is a splendid way of helping blind children to be familiar with door catches and fastenings and may perhaps avoid the frightening experience of them shutting themselves in the toilet and not knowing how to handle the lock. It is also very useful for children who have difficulty with door knobs or bolts, but is not recommended for children who need to be restricted, and for whom bolts and catches must remain a mystery for as long as possible! The board can be made to meet individual requirements and catches fitted to suit. The original Open Sesame Board was made for my little blind friend and consisted of a large sheet of wood about 3' x 2' which could be propped against the wall or used on a table top. Six oblongs were cut out of the wood and a small box was made behind each hole. The oblongs were fitted back on hinges as doors to the little boxes and each one closed in a different way—with a bolt, handle, key, suitcase catch, hook, or button catch like the one on the rabbit hutch. A simpler version can be made with only four doors with no boxes behind them. This can be laid on a table and a picture put behind each door (an old Christmas Card will do). When the child opens the door he will find the picture. He can then choose another picture to hide away for the next person to find.

Feely Box

This has been used most successfully with easily distracted children, such as a young deaf boy excluded from school because of behaviour problems, and it has

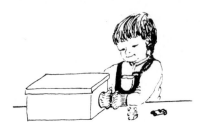

encouraged children with speech problems to talk.

It consists of a shoe box with a hole cut in one end and the leg of an old sock fitted to this. The child pushes his hand down the sock and through the hole in the end of the box to discover what is hidden in it. This mystery object can be a complete surprise and he must identify it by feel before taking off the lid of the box or pulling the object out through the sock to see if he has guessed correctly. Alternatively he can put three or four objects into the box, having a good look at them as he does so, and then he can be asked to poke his hand through the sock and feel around in the box to find the square thing, or the round thing etc. It is a good toy for encouraging a child to use touch, sight and speech and has been used very successfully to help children identify by feel natural objects such as pebbles, shells, feathers, conkers, acorns and fir cones.

Tins on a Post

This is an excellent stacking toy for the very young. It is not suitable for older retarded children who may still need this kind of toy as they could possibly crush the tins and so make them dangerous.

Firmly fix a length of broom handle, about 6″ long, into a wooden base about 6″ square by drilling a hole and gluing it in. This makes a good holder for the tins, but is *not essential* to the success of the toy. Collect a selection of food tins of different heights and diameters. Carefully remove the top *and bottom* with a rotary tin opener which should turn the edges in safely. Run your finger gently round each rim to check for any sharpness. Only keep tins which are perfectly smooth and safe. Paint the outsides of the tins with Humbrol enamel. The child can then stack them on the post and because they are all round they can be put on in any order and will always fit! They will nest equally well without the post.

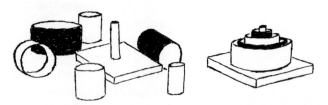

An Easily Made Fishing Game for Older Children

Cut out several fish shapes from thin cardboard (plain post cards will do). Fix paper clips in the position of the eyes. The sort with little tabs which bend back, called daisy clips, are the best. It is safest to sandwich two fish shapes together with these tabs buried between the layers of cardboard. Make a fishing rod from a length of dowel or an old washing up mop handle and tie a magnet to the end of the line. Make sure the magnet is strong enough to lift the fish. Round industrial magnets sold at tool shops are best. Put the cardboard fish in a large bowl and let the child catch them with he rod, line and magnet. To make the game more interesting the fish can be numbered on their undersides, two children can take it in turns to fish and scores can be kept.

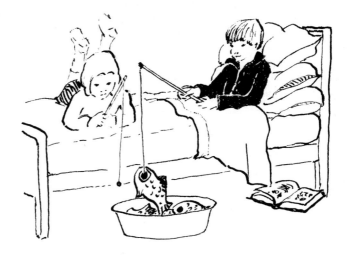

BOOK LIST

Clay
Fun With Clay
G. C. Payne   Kaye and Ward 1967
Simple processes clearly explained.
The Young Potter
Denys Van Baker   Kaye and Ward 1963
How to use clay. Ideas for beginners.

Collage
Fun With Collage
Jan Beaney   Kaye and Ward 1970

Many ideas for using paper, textiles, egg boxes etc.
Seed Picture Making
Roger and Glenda Marsh   Blandford Press
Many ideas are possible for handicapped children if other materials are used eg. butterbeans instead of peas, or perhaps pebbles, bottletops, buttons etc.
Let's Make a Mosaic
June Tanner   Angus and Robertson 1968
How to do it using seeds, wood and nails, tiles, pebbles etc. Suggestions for the practical application of these techniques.

Decorations
Making Decorations
Elizabeth Gundry   Piccolo 1974
How to Make Decorations
Michael Kingsley Skinner   Studio Vista 1974
Lots of Fun to Make Decorations
Collette Lamarque   Collins 1973

Needlework
Make it from Felt
Phyllis Chappell   Evans Bros. 1974
My Learn to Sew Book
Janet Barber   Hamlyn 1971
How to Sew Presents from Scraps
Gillian Lockwood   Studio Vista 1974
Lots of Fun to Make a Gift
Compiled from ideas from Golden Hands   Collins 1971
Clear colourful instructions. Some articles are easier to make than others, so this book could be suitable for a wide age range.

Miscellaneous
Paper Scissors and Paste
Pipe Cleaner Figures
Both in the Leisure Craft Series   Burns and Oates Ltd.
Suitable for older children.
Fun to Make Book
More Fun to Make Book
Both by Collette Lamarque   Collins
Games to Make and Play
Brian Edwards   Purnell 1974

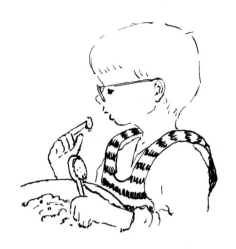

4 Making the most of TASTE

This chapter is concerned with tasting games and activities which involve playing with food. It is impossible to enter a toy shop and ask for a tasty toy. Perhaps the nearest thing would be sweets in a fancy package, or a chocolate flavoured bone for a puppy! However, this does not mean that the sense of taste should be overlooked as a potential source of fun. For some severely disabled children using the tongue may be their best, and perhaps their only, way of discovering more about their environment and finding enjoyment from sensation. Stimulation at this level may not be real 'play', but it could be a form of pleasure and as such should not be disregarded by anyone caring for such children.

LEARNING TO BE SELECTIVE

Some children who normally enjoy their food may not want to stop eating once the meal is over. The problem can then be to try to prevent them from being like an ostrich, sampling everything within reach — even those things which are unpleasant or dangerous. These children are still playing at the baby stage when everything that can be grasped is explored for shape and texture by the mouth and lips first, rather than by the fingers. They are like an adventurous crawler who will try eating mud, coal, or even potato peelings, seeming to find them all delicious. Parents usually notice that a baby's mouth is the first thing to bring him pleasure. With it he can satisfy his hunger and enjoy the comfortable feeling of wellbeing. As he grows bigger, like the baby in the pram described in earlier chapters, he will be able to see, hear, and feel with his hands and feet, but he will still like to do plenty of exploring with his mouth. At first he will be discovering tastes and textures without discriminating between them. Gradually he will learn to be selective, showing a preference for some of them and a strong objection to others.

For the majority of children taste takes its place with all the other senses in helping to enrich daily living, but some handicapped children need to be helped to be aware of it, just as they need to be encouraged in the use of their other senses and the following pages may suggest ways of making the most of taste.

FUN WITH FOOD

Parents of faddy children know that serving a meal in a surprise way, or involving a child in its preparation can often help to make food more attractive. Play can turn meal times into something to look forward to instead of a dreaded endless battle of wills.

If you have time and inclination, you can think up many ways of playing with food and letting your child help you; decorating food is perhaps the most obvious. For example, faces can be made with the ingredients of a salad, perhaps using watercress for curly hair, hard boiled egg slices for eyes (if the yoke is not central you can have saucy eyes looking sideways, or horrific squints), tomato slices for rosy cheeks, a radish for a mouth, a droopy moustache from cress and lettuce to make a collar.

Apple or orange segments can be arranged into patterns or flowers. Grapes cut in half with the pips removed make good centres for these. Shapes can be cut out of a slice of cheese. A child can help here, using a blunt knife and, of course, eating the offcuts. Squares of processed cheese are excellent for this and are just the right size for cutting into a house shape with a door and windows and a pitched roof. The piece cut out for the door can make the chimney pots.

Cookery books and magazines are full of good ideas, especially if you consult the children's party pages, and some of the food advertisements.

SOME GROUP GAMES
INVOLVING FOOD AND TASTE

Hocus Pocus

This game was taught to me by a Swiss friend who worked in a children's hospital, and I suspect she invented it. It can become a firm favourite with all young children who are mature enough to take turns. It includes a ritual sentence and the eating of sweets, and every player can be a winner. It is most successful when played with a small group so that turns come round quite quickly. Imagine a little bunch of children gathered round a leader who has in her lap a plate and a bag of small sweets. One child is chosen to hide his eyes in the corner of the room. The leader puts three sweets on the plate, perhaps a green, a red and an orange one. The children gathered round the plate chant 'Hocus Pocus, don't eat ME'. At 'me' the leader points to one of the sweets, say the red one, and that has now become 'magic'. The chosen child comes out of his corner and tries to guess which is the magic sweet. If he points to the green or orange ones he may eat those, but if he points to the 'magic' red one he may eat that, but *no more!* Whatever his choice he is certain to have at least one sweet and if he is lucky he may have two or even three if he manages to pick the 'magic' one last. The children watching enjoy seeing the chosen child make his guess, and will clap all the lucky guesses and groan when the 'magic' one is taken. At the end of the game it is time to share out the remainder of the sweets!

For overweight children or those who should not have sugar this game can be played equally well with small pieces of fruit or even with different shaped breakfast cereals.

Shop Treasure Hunt

This game is a 'must' at all our family birthday parties.

The 'treasure' is exchanged for small sweets at the 'shop' but peanuts, crisps, sugar puffs or raisins could be used equally well. The 'treasure' is hidden all over the house. Butter beans are suitable but buttons or short lengths of wool or even grains of rice if you want to make the game really hard, could be used equally well. One child is shop keeper and in charge of the sweet stall. The rest search for the treasure. There is an agreed rate of exchange e.g. 1 bean = 1 sweet, or you can have more complicated bartering like 1 bean = 1 round Dolly mixture, 1 bean = 2 peanuts. You make up the rules to suit the age and ability of the players! Everyone has a turn at being shopkeeper and the beans can be surreptitiously rehidden for as long as the shop supply lasts. It is a good idea to issue the stock for the shop by degrees as some shop keepers have been known to be very hungry!

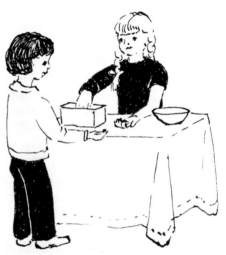

Yummy Yum

This is a tasting game popular at parties for older children who can write. Each child is blindfolded, then given a plate containing small pieces of favourite foods. These might include a peanut, a raisin, a slice of apple, banana and cucumber, a Dolly mixture or other small sweet, a sugar lump, a tiny biscuit, etc. When each plate has been consumed blindfolds are removed and the children make a list of as many of the tastes as they can remember. This game can easily be simplified and played at meal times. The child who needs feeding closes his eyes and says what food is presented to him with each spoonful. This also helps him to associate the name of the food with its taste.

ACTIVITIES INVOLVING FOOD AND TASTE

Growing a Cress Hedgehog

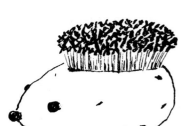

You will need:-
- A Potato
- A teaspoon
- 4 dead matchsticks
- A little cotton wool
- Some cress seeds

Choose a potato which is roughly the shape of a hedgehog and about the size of a serving spoon. Scoop out a hollow with the teaspoon in the middle of the top where you think the prickles should grow. Take the burnt heads off the matches and poke two into the front of the potato to make the eyes, and one at the very front to be the nose. Poke the matchsticks in the bottom of the potato to make the hedgehog's legs. Fill the scooped out top with cotton wool and damp this well. Sprinkle liberally with cress seeds. Mustard seeds grow more quickly but most children prefer the milder tasting cress. Stand the hedgehog in a light warm place where he can be watched and admired. Water him daily and before a week is up he should have a splendid crop of cress growing on his back. This can be 'harvested', washed and eaten with great ceremony.

Making Butter

You will need:-
- A glass jar with a firmly fitting screw top, preferably with a wide neck, such as a honey jar
- The top of the milk
- A pinch of salt
- A knife
- Plain biscuits to spread the butter on.

Making butter can be a tedious process but is fun if several children take turns at shaking. As a glass jar is involved supervision is necessary. The container must be transparent so that the butter can be seen forming. Butter made in a plastic Squash bottle could be safer, but it is difficult to get the butter out through the narrow neck.

The cream from the top of the milk and a pinch of salt are put into the jar and the lid firmly screwed on. The children can sit in a circle and take it in turns to shake. Perhaps the other children can do ten or twenty claps all together so that the shaking time is fairly rationed out. At first the milk becomes bubbly but gradually little blobs of cream collect together on the surface and these finally form one big lump. Spread this on the biscuits and have a feast!

Teddy Bears' Picnics or Dolls' Tea Parties

These are a most satisfying occupation for any child handicapped or not and are enjoyed even more if dressing up is included. If the family has just celebrated a birthday the remains of the candles can be put on a little cake and used for a doll (or a teddy) who is the new 'birthday child'. This doll will need help to blow out the candles and this can provide practice for a child who finds breath control hard.

I remember a very wet afternoon when our family morale was definitely in need of an uplift. We decided it was Big Ted's birthday. Every doll and stuffed animal in

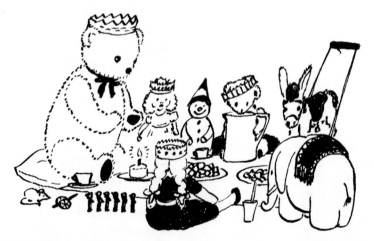

the house was collected and arranged on cushions in a large circle round the table cloth which was spread on the floor. The big toys propped up the little ones and everyone was dressed in party best. Paper crowns were hastily made from long strips of coloured paper cut with pinking shears and decorated with felt pen. Table napkins were made from paper tissues. The party guests obligingly listened to records while the feast was prepared. This consisted of little star biscuits, tiny Marmite or paste sandwiches about 1" square, Mini Choc Rolls cut into slices, new carrot sticks, raisins and peanuts—all these vanished during the course of the game!

Incidentally this is a wonderful way to coax a convalescent to eat without seeming to make a fuss. One mother I know adds to the fun of dolls' tea parties by putting a few drops of food colouring in the milk which is poured from the toy tea pot.

Jam Tarts

'Tarts for tea!' This was the cry sometimes heard on Friday afternoons at a hospital school in London. The children were mostly up and about and some would have gone home for the weekend so a morale raiser for those left behind was obviously needed. The cooking and preparation was done methodically and thoroughly. The children's finger nails, hands and wrists were happily scrubbed, table tops were scoured and the few bed children draped with protective plastic sheeting. Then came the measuring out and the mixing up. Sometimes this was done in a big bowl with everyone taking their turn at mixing the flour and fat until they looked like the 'breadcrumbs' described in cookery books. When there were a few children each one could rub in his own. Next came the ceremonial lighting of the ward oven to heat (stand well back there!) and the rolling and cutting of the pastry and the big decision whether to fill the tarts with lemon curd or strawberry jam. While the tarts were baked the grand clear up began. If this was accomplished with speed and efficiency there would be time for a game of Hocus Pocus (see page 121). Then everyone enjoyed a tart for tea and some were saved for the evening visitors.

RECIPES WHICH DO NOT REQUIRE COOKING

Open Sandwiches

(Not good for messy eaters as the toppings tend to fall off.)

Start with a slab of something plain like bread, toast or roll. Butter this and add your own favourite toppings from this list of suggestions:- cheese, egg, sardine, liver sausage or Marmite. Add lettuce, cress, tomato or watercress. For sweet toppings—honey and dates or jam and cream cheese are popular. A few strawberries will go a long way if sliced and arranged on fairly thick fingers of bread and sprinkled with sugar.

Sandwich Fillings

These can be made 'according to taste'. All the child needs to do is to mash everything together with a fork in a deep basin, so that all the ingredients combine to make a fairly stiff spread. Quantities have been kept vague on purpose. If a child does not like salad cream leave this out and add more tomato, or the other way round. A little butter can always be added to make a spread softer but mix this in a very small amount at a time in case the spread suddenly becomes too soft and greasy.

Meat Spread

You will need:-
A small tin of corned beef or meat loaf
Tomatoes or tomato purée
Salad cream
A pinch of salt and a shake of pepper
Chop up the meat so that it will mash more easily. Skin the tomatoes. (Pop them into hot water for a short while. This will soften the skin of the tomato, cooking it a little, and it will then peel off easily). Add a small amount of tomato, salad cream and salt and pepper. With the fork mash the mixture until it is well mixed, gradually adding more tomato and salad cream until the concoction is smooth enough to spread.

Cheese and Tomato Spread

You will need:-
Grated cheese
A teaspoonful of chutney
About two tomatoes
A pinch of salt and a shake of pepper
Grate the cheese, (a Multi Mouli Grater is safe for children to use—they cannot hurt their knuckles on the cutting surface which is enclosed in a plastic case) add the chutney, chop up some skinned tomato and add it

gradually until the mixture is soft enough to spread.

Egg and Cheese Spread

You will need:-
Hard boiled egg
Some grated cheese
A little butter
Salad cream
A pinch of salt and a shake of pepper
Chop up the egg and add all the other ingredients, mashing them up until they are well mixed.

Making Instant Whip

Do this according to the directions on the packet. Children love to feel the liquid thickening as they mix, and this is 'cooking' which young blind children can enjoy. The finished whip can be spooned into small dishes to make individual portions for all the family, and this gives practice in being careful not to spill.

If a child needs encouragement to use both hands he can use a sieve and a rotary whisk to make this pudding. The Instant Whip powder can be rubbed through a sieve with the back of a spoon. The sieve can be balanced across the top of the bowl with the milk in, but it will need steadying while the powder is pushed through, and if the bowl is not very deep it will have to be held clear of the milk. All this needs considerable skill. For children with sufficient strength and hand control, using a rotary whisk can be both a challenge and great fun. One hand must grasp the top·handle to hold the whisk steady and upright while the other hand turns the wheel to rotate the blades—almost as hard for some as trying to rub your tummy and pat your head! Energetic children tend to spatter the Instant Whip in all directions so standing the mixing bowl in the sink can save some of the mess.

Gooseberry Fool

You will need:-
a tin of gooseberrys (or fresh stewed ones)
some custard, tinned or freshly made
a little castor sugar
Whisk all of these together until they are well blended and pour the mixture into individual glasses. Decorate with half a glacé cherry and chill.

This is another recipe requiring a rotary hand whisk.

Provide a deep bowl or an enthusiastic cook might spray the mixture everywhere.

SWEETS WHICH DO NOT REQUIRE COOKING

Fondant Creams

Icing sugar and a *very little* white of egg mixed together make a firm dough which can be moulded into shapes and decorated with pieces of glacé cherries or edible little silver balls. You can get variety by adding a few drops of colour or flavouring, eg, peppermint essence, coffee essence (which can be made by dissolving a teaspoonful of instant coffee in a very little boiling water), or lemon juice to the egg white before you mix it in. If the icing sugar is lumpy it should be crushed with a rolling pin and sieved.

An easy way for a child to separate the white of an egg from the yolk is to break the egg onto a plate, hold an egg cup over the yolk and slide the white off the plate into a basin.

The dough can be rolled out and cut into shapes, or moulded by hand.

The finished sweets must be laid to dry on some greaseproof paper which has been sprinkled with icing sugar.

Stuffed Dates

Remove the stone from each date, make a small sausage of fondant cream about the same size as the stone and pop this inside the date. Top with a piece of walnut.

Coconut Ice

You will need—
    8 oz. dessicated coconut
    8 oz. icing sugar
    a small tin of *sweetened* condensed
    milk, (about two tablespoons)
Mix these together to make a stiff dough, adding the condensed milk very gradually. If you want pink coconut ice add cochineal to the condensed milk before

you stir it into the dry ingredients. Press the mixture into a tin which has been sprinkled with icing sugar and leave it to set.

These sweets are all quite easy to prepare. They can be a good present for a child to make for someone's birthday or for Christmas.

MAKING THE MOST OF THE KITCHEN

Apart from a few games and Big Ted's birthday party all the activities in this chapter could have taken place in the kitchen. This room is often the hub of family life while the children are young. Here it is busy and companionable. It is the place where Mum can usually be found for it is her workshop and storeroom rolled into one. It is worthwhile arranging the kitchen so that it is possible for children to play there safely.

The kitchen has many advantages as a play area. It has an easily cleaned floor, table space for quiet games, running water and a stock of perfect toys. Everyone knows the strongest and noisiest drums are made from a saucepan and a wooden spoon, and it is much more fun to unscrew the lids from real pots than to play with toy plastic ones. The tools of the kitchen are big and strong, shiny and colourful. Though some are dangerous and unsuitable for play, others are ideal toys. Of course there are moments such as jam making days and dishing up time when children, for their own protection, must be firmly excluded from, or confined to a safe area of the kitchen, but at other times this room can be the best possible place for a mother and child to enjoy each other's company. Cupboards can be rearranged to make them safe from busy fingers, doors can be tied up or barricaded with a table, low shelves can be filled with saucepans and baking tins while dangerous things and fragile glass bottles and jars are stored safely out of reach. A guard rail fitted to the cooker is a good safety device, and all saucepan handles must always be turned away from the front of the stove to prevent children from grasping them and pulling the scalding contents over themselves.

The following descriptions of 'kitchen play' show how some severely handicapped children can be amused happily and usefully while the essential work of running the household continues.

Watching Mummy Work

Mrs A. has waved her family off to school and is about to tackle the breakfast dishes. Baby Susan aged 6 months is believed to be severely deaf. She has been bathed and fed and now feels like some fun before it is time for her nap. She is kicking happily in her Baby Relax which is on the floor but Mrs A. realises this activity gives her a very limited view and will soon bore her. She lifts the Baby Relax to the far corner of her large draining board, wedges it securely and hands Susan an old spoon to wave about, suck and bang on the draining board. Then she turns her attention to the dishes. As soon as the taps are turned on Susan abandons her spoon for this fascinating sight. The streams of water gush out. She is attracted by the silvery flow and watches intently as the water splashes in the basin. She does not hear the sound of the water but does she notice that one stream of water is steamy? Perhaps not, but she is obviously concentrating hard and thoroughly enjoying this new experience. Her Mother puts the detergent in the basin and realises that the bottle is nearly empty. She swishes a little water round inside the bottle and skilfully squeezes it to make it blow a stream of little bubbles. Susan is delighted and they both laugh as they share the joke. Mrs A. washes the bottle properly and puts it aside to dry. It will make a splendid squeezing toy for Susan later on. She can puff the air out of the top, or her big sister will find a few small pebbles to put inside to turn it into a shaker for her. The stopper will be firmly glued on with a dab of polystyrene cement in case she should decide to chew it.

Now the washing up begins and Susan is fascinated by all the shapes and colours which are fished out of the steaming bowl. Mrs A. hands her a plastic egg cup to examine. This soon lands on the floor and she is given a teaspoon still warm from the bowl of suds. Does she think 'That's curious—the spoon I had just now was

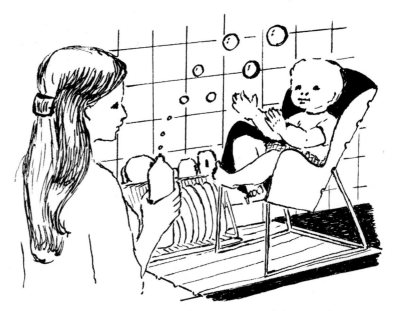

cold and soothing to my hot gums—this one is warm and tastes funny!' Of course she cannot express herself in so many words but in time she will begin to notice all those little things that are so familiar to us that we don't even bother to think about them. When she is older Mrs A. will give her the tea spoons to sort from the cereal spoons and she will stack up the plastic dishes and plates. She will be enjoying the ever popular game of 'Let's pretend to be Mummy', and learning without knowing it about size and shape and weight.

Playing at the Sink

Mrs B. is about to tackle a very grubby wash. The family had a picnic on the Common yesterday and all that tree climbing and playing Commandos has left the tee shirts and jeans in a very sorry state. Gareth is a Mongol of eight who has an extra holiday from school today and he is lonely while his brothers are away. Mrs B. decides to make a pie for supper before she tackles the washing, but she needs to amuse Gareth while she works. She looks at the pile of washing and decides that nothing could possibly make it worse, so today is the ideal day for a 'water frolic'. She fetches a little stool and places it in front of the sink. She spreads the dirty washing on the floor all round the stool to mop up the inevitable flood. She half fills the sink with tepid water. Luckily the

131

day is very warm so Gareth can remove his shoes and socks. Wearing a plastic apron of his Mother's and very little else he climbs on the stool, full of anticipation for the delights to come. His Mother gives him a colander and he spends several minutes pressing it into the water, watching the water well up through the holes until it is full, then lifting it up with both hands to see the water gush out again. Meanwhile Mrs B. assembles the ingredients for her pie. The colander begins to lose its appeal and any moment it will be held over the dirty washing to make a thunder shower as the water floods through the holes. Mrs B. has an instinct for such things and before removing the colander hands Gareth a favourite toy which is an old detergent bottle which has been cut about 2'' from the top and the stopper removed so that it makes a funnel. He has learnt to put a finger over the stopper hole while he fills the funnel with a spoon. This is a useful exercise for him and he

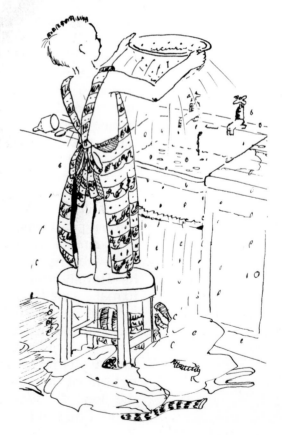

concentrates hard to keep the spoon level while he scoops the water from the basin to the funnel. Then comes the joyous moment when the funnel is full and he must take his finger away to release the water. He holds it high so that the water will have a long drop. He slightly tilts the funnel towards himself and is slow to remove his finger so that most of the water runs down his arm to drip off the end of his elbow onto the floor. Luckily the grubby clothes absorb it all. With infinite patience Gareth starts to refill the funnel with his spoon. When he tires of this his Mother gives him some scraps of Polystyrene tile left over from a decorating job. Gareth spends some time trying to force these to sink. However often he pokes them to the bottom of the basin he discovers that as soon as he takes his finger away they bob up to the surface again. Does he realise that the spoon he was using will never float and that he has been handling two very interesting substances?

Mrs B. has finished her pie and saved the pastry offcuts for Gareth to play with later. She looks at the Polystyrene and has a brainwave. She reaches in the drawer for an old paper bag and a cocktail stick. She tears a little sail from the bag and turns the stick into a tiny mast. She shows Gareth the sharp pointed ends and warns him not to touch them. She fixes the mast and sail to a piece of polystyrene to make a crude boat. She shows Gareth how to blow gently and make the boat sail across the sink. With his enlarged tongue he finds this difficult but is delighted when he achieves a little success. Suddenly he tires of the whole game, snatches out the plug and chuckles with delight as the little boat whirls madly round the plughole. His Mother turns her attention to the grubby washing while Gareth tries his hand with the pastry scraps.

JUST BEING COMPANIONABLE

Mrs C. has Mary home for the week-end. Her husband has taken lively little Peter to 'help' to do the shopping and after lunch uncle and aunty and two little cousins will be coming to tea. Mary lies on her mattress out of the draught, in the corner of the kitchen. She is eleven years old, and severely mentally retarded. Her body is stiff, she has difficulty in focusing her eyes and only has very limited movement in her left arm and hand. She has grown too tall to fit on the cot mattress so her feet are supported on a cushion. After lunch she will lie on the couch or sit propped up in her chair so that she can be included in the tea party. Usually she lives at the Subnormality hospital about five miles away where her parents visit her as often as they can. Every other week-end she comes home. Today her mother has moved the breakfast stools into the hall and pushed the table to one side so that Mary can watch her prepare the lunch and tea. Just now Mary is lying on her right side so that her 'good' left arm is free to move to the best

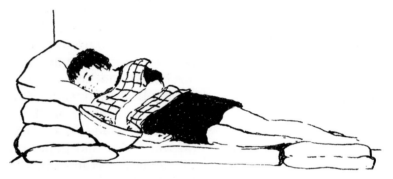

advantage. Every time Mrs C. passes her she shakes her hand and Mary smiles. Mrs C, is about to mix a cake, so she ties a piece of string across Mary's corner and hangs up a new baby's rattle she has just bought. It is plastic and is like a small hand mirror with a reflective surface one side and a few seeds between the front and back which make a pleasant soft sound when shaken. Mary clenches her fist and punches the rattle making it swing on its string. She enjoys the noise and the reflected light from the mirror. Now she seems to have forgotten all about it. Her mother passes and shakes hands. Mary notices the mirror again. She gives it another punch, hitting it off centre so that it revolves as it swings. She makes little gurgling sounds of happiness as she watches the mirror side come and go.

Now the cake is ready for the oven and Mrs C. clears away all the paraphanalia. She is about to wash out the mixing bowl when she remembers Mary. She tucks a tea towel under her chin, rolls up her left sleeve, props the basin at the right angle and guides Mary's fist as she wipes it round the bowl, and helps her suck off the delicious cake mixture. The smell of the baking cake fills the kitchen as Mrs C. starts to clean Mary and the mixing bowl.

BOOK LIST

Fruit and Vegetable Figures
Leisure Craft Series   Burns and Oates Ltd.
Mother's Help
Ed. Susan Dickinson   Collins 1972
(Has an excellent chapter on cookery for playgroups. Recipes involve using a cooker).
345 Very First Cook Book
Iris Grender   Kiddicraft 1973
Look I Can Cook
Angela Burdick   Octopus 1972
Cooking is Easy When You Know How
Isabelle Barrett   Golden Hands Junior 1974
My Round the Year Cook Book
Susan Conner   Nelson Young World 1974
The Nursery Rhyme Cookery Books
R. H. S. Publications 1973
The Play and Cook Book
Marguerite Pattern   Collins 1973
Floury Fingers
Celia H Hinde   Faber 1962
The Pooh Cook Book
Katie Stewart   Methuen   1971
Let's Have a Party
Maureen Roffey   The Bodley Head 1974
Ideas for invitations, decorations, games, food, and take home presents.

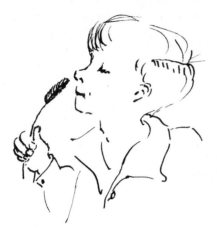

5 Making the most of SMELL

The sense of smell is perhaps the least *obviously* stimulating and useful of all the five senses, but it can give great pleasure, and to children who lack efficient sight it is also extremely useful as a mobility aid. Imagine you know these two children. Peter is seven and is severely subnormal. The greater part of his life has been spent in his hospital cot. If a few drops of perfume are sprinkled on his pillow he will make a big effort to turn his head to enjoy the smell. Mark is ten and attends a school for the blind. During the holidays he often shops for his mother and always manages successfully. He has never been known to confuse the butcher's shop for the baker's for he can confidently distinguish them by smell. He had learnt to trust his nose to confirm all the information he can receive through his ears and fingers. Between these two children with their special problems lies the vast army of handicapped children, each one with his own personal difficulties. For all of them life can be enriched if they make the most of every sense, and that means including the sense of smell.

LEARNING TO SMELL

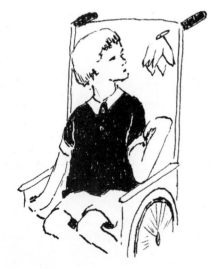

We are aware when a baby has learnt to focus because we see him stare at something that interests him, or he will look into our eyes and smile back at us. We know he is aware of sound when there is a noise behind him and

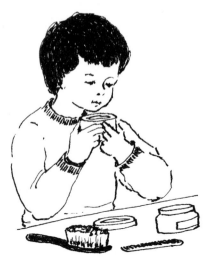

he turns his head to investigate. His delight in his sense of touch is obvious when his fat little fingers start to grasp and poke and stroke all the interesting textures he finds. At mealtimes he makes it perfectly clear that some tastes please him more than others, but it seems as though a conscious sense of smell takes a little longer to unfold. If you hand a flower to a young child and invite him to smell it he will probably wrinkle up his nose but instead of sniffing will snort or snuffle. At this stage he is likely to have problems blowing out his birthday candles too, so perhaps he just lacks control over his breathing. By the time he has become mobile and increasingly skillful with his hands he may discover that ecstatic experience of unscrewing the lids from his mother's cosmetic jars and be discovered sniffing appreciatively at their pleasing perfumes. As he grows older smells will have certain associations and will help to enrich his memories and perhaps even warn him of danger. Every adult has made his own catalogue of smells built up over the years and many of these will have been discovered in childhood and remembered ever since. Perhaps the smell of new leather shoes is associated with stiff shiny sandals on the first day of the summer term, or the smell of mud flats at low tide is a reminder of a happy holiday. When we think about smells we realise we all have our own particular likes and dislikes, just as we do with sights, sounds, feels and tastes, but unless we have the opportunity to explore and experiment we may never discover what we like.

HELPING HANDICAPPED CHILDREN TO ENJOY THE SENSE OF SMELL

The mobile child who is able to explore, though he may be deaf or blind, can reach for things he wants to examine. The physically handicapped child may be severely restricted by his disability and have to rely on others to keep him supplied with interesting objects to investigate and smell. Slow-learners may be just incurious. Though an exciting smell may be within their reach they may need to have their attention directed

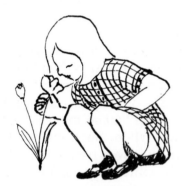

towards it before they will seem to take any notice. Some emotionally disturbed children may smell everything they handle but often this action does not seem to have any particular significance. It can be just part of a ritual. How can all these children be helped to develop and enjoy the sense of smell? Parents who hope to solve the problem by visiting a toy shop will find there are scarcely any smelly toys available. Smells are such transitory things, literally carried away by the wind, that any manufacturer, no matter how enterprising, would be hard put to it to add a universally acceptable and long lasting one to his product. This means that those of us who are concerned with the play needs of handicapped children must make an effort to think about introducing smells into play, just as we provide colour, sound and texture. If smelly toys are in short supply we must make use of activities and games which include different perfumes—some well-tried ones are described in this chapter—but perhaps the richest source of stimulating smells is the child's own environment. One imaginative teacher takes her severely handicapped children to lie in the long grass at the end of their ward garden. Imagine how delightful it must be to be surrounded by the waving grasses and to smell the warm earth and the hay—surely a pleasant change from the smell of cotton sheets and soap suds. In the winter this same teacher sometimes buys a packet of dried herbs from the supermarket and puts a few leaves in a little bag made from an old curtain and hangs it near to a child. He might otherwise never have the chance to smell mint or bay leaves or basil. A mother who uses our Toy Library borrowed the pastry set and made a batch of play pastry for her child to roll out and cut. To begin with he was not at all interested, but knowing he liked the smell of peppermint she added a few drops of essence to the dough. From then on he played with it happily, and enjoyed squeezing, prodding and rolling it, finally chopping it into little pieces with a plastic paper knife.

It takes imagination to think of such ways of stimulating children but it is a skill that can be developed. Even the everyday experience of going shopping can be either a dull chore or an exciting outing of discovery. Imagine you can watch the mothers in the two following situations and draw your own conclusions as to whose child you would rather be!

Mrs A is going shopping with Peter who is four years old and blind. She is in a hurry today because her friend is coming to tea and she has had a hindering morning. The shops are not far away, but to save time she pops Peter in the push chair and walks there as quickly as possible, hurrying over her selection of food at the supermarket and remembering the bottle of white spirit she has promised to buy for her husband. On the way home her plastic shopping bag is in danger of splitting with the weight of all her purchases so she gives the white spirit and a bottle of lemonade to Peter to hold, one in each arm, as he sits in the push chair. When she reaches home she takes them from him and Peter hears her put them on the kitchen table with the other shopping. She turns her attention to helping Peter with his coat and gloves, answers the 'phone and puts the push chair away. The front door bell rings. It is the milkman calling to be paid. Meanwhile Peter fancies a drink of lemonade. He knows the bottle is on the table. He remembers it is tall and heavy because he nursed it all the way home. Confidently he reaches on the shelf for his mug and places it on the draining board. He takes the nearest bottle, unscrews the lid, and begins to pour. Luckily Mrs A. returns to the kitchen at that moment so disaster is averted!

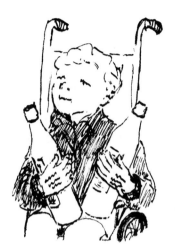

Mrs B. is also going shopping, taking with her four year old Lucy (who is blind) and the baby. Her shopping list is not long today; just white spirit, lemonade, coffee, toilet soap, fish and some parsley for the sauce. Lucy walks briskly along, holding on to the handle of the pram. She knows when she is nearly at the end of her road because the gentleman who lives in the last house has planted an evergreen hedge and this has a special smell and tickles her fingers as she drags them through the young branches. The gentleman is busy gardening. She can hear his shears cutting the grass border on the other side of the hedge. He calls a greeting and the shopping expedition is diverted through the front gate. He wants to show Lucy how well his herb garden is growing so they all go round to the side of the house.

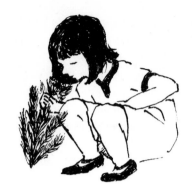

Here, Lucy who can already identify sage, parsley and mint, is delighted to examine a little bush of rosemary, crushing a few leaves between her fingers to increase the smell. A few moments later they go on their way, Mrs B. with a bag of parsley for the sauce and Lucy with a little posy of herbs to plant in a saucer garden when she reaches home. Further down the street they pause to make way for the delivery man who is carrying a big wooden tray full of freshly made rolls into the baker's shop. They smell so good Mrs B. and Lucy decide to buy some. Later, in the supermarket, Lucy pushes the trolley to the corner where the coffee grinder is kept. Mrs B. selects the beans she wants, takes one out and gives it to Lucy to play with while the others are being ground. Before she seals down the bag she gives Lucy the opportunity to feel the soft coffee powder and smell its particular fragrance. Now to buy the toilet soap. There is plenty of chance to sniff and compare here and Lucy is allowed to chose the one she likes best. Mrs B. then gropes in the freezer for the fish and adds the bottle of lemonade to the contents of Lucy's trolley. They make for the check out nearest the greengrocery shelves. Many of the trays for the fruit and vegetables are at the edge of the shelf, just level with Lucy's nose, and without touching them she can slide along the edge of the counter and try to identify them by smell. Here are the apples, oranges and bananas. Next come cauliflower, onions and earthy potatoes. Each time they play this game Lucy becomes more sure of the answers. They leave the supermarket and go to the ironmongers. They find the manager arranging a new delivery of candles. He accidently drops one. Quickly Lucy feels for it and holds it up for him. She is enjoying the sensation of the wax against her hot fingers which are rapidly exploring this fascinating object with its little tail of string. The lady who buys that candle may well wonder why it has tiny grooves up one side. Only Lucy will know they are where she poked her thumb nail in! Mrs B. buys the white spirit. The manager turns to help another customer and while they wait to pay, Mrs B. realises she has just bought something potentially dangerous of which Lucy has so far had no experience. She tells her about the white spirit and why daddy will need it to clean his paint brushes. She lets her examine the bottle and then carefully removes the stopper so that she can smell the dangerous liquid. She pays for it and makes a great fuss, placing it at the foot of the pram where baby cannot possibly reach it. The shopping now done, Mrs B. turns the pram towards home, a nice cup of coffee, new bread rolls and a refreshing drink of lemonade for Lucy.

There are several lessons to be learnt from these two shopping expeditions. Mrs A. in her understandable hurry to complete the trip as quickly as possible, has done nothing to increase Peter's knowledge of his environment. All he has gained from this particular outing is a breath of fresh air. Mrs B. has realised the need to encourage Lucy's awareness of smells and finds several opportunities during the walk to make use of this skill. Lucy can already identify by smell the neighbour's hedge, the baker's shop and various departments of the supermarket. She has been taught the new smell and the name of the herb rosemary, she has enjoyed sniffing at the coffee and the soaps, and the guessing game with the fruit and vegetables. She has also learnt to be warned of danger by learning to identify by smell the poisonous white spirit. This early training in using her nose will help to give her valuable independence so that she will be able to take herself unaccompanied on similar shopping expeditions when she is older. Meanwhile this particular walk has increased both her vocabulary and her self confidence.

USING SMELLS FOR FUN

It is easy to go around the house and find many things which may well be heading for the dustbin that could first be used as splendid toys to stimulate the sense of smell. An *EMPTY* talcum powder tin is a good example. It has an attractive shape and colour, and a lingering perfume most babies love. Opening and closing the holes is fun for toddlers with strong fingers. The ends of cakes of toilet soap can be dissolved in hot water to make smelly bubble mixture, or you can use a perfumed detergent. A few drops of glycerine added to the bubble mixture will make much tougher bubbles, and a small amount of mixture in a cup will blow into an impressive mound of bubbles reaching very near the child's nose so that he cannot fail to smell it!

Older children enjoy squeezing the bulb of an old empty scent spray, and these can sometimes be bought very cheaply at jumble sales. (Beware of letting children play with the modern equivalent—aerosol cans. A child who cannot read and who is allowed to use an air freshener cannot be expected to recognise the difference between that can and one containing oven cleaner or touch-up paint.) A substitute puffing scent spray can be made very quickly from an empty plastic detergent bottle. Take off the nozzle, wash it, and rinse out the bottle to remove all trace of the detergent smell. Put in any smelly substance your child would enjoy—there are many suggested in this chapter. One small girl spent a happy afternoon filling a plastic puffer with fallen rose petals. The final result was not entirely satisfactory; the petals tended to clog the air jet, but she had thoroughly enjoyed herself experimenting! Once you have put in the smell replace the nozzle. If this toy has been made for an older child and there is any danger of his being able to remove the top be careful to use very safe materials to provide the smell. You can also stick the nozzle on with a dab of quick drying polystyrene cement (used for making up plastic model kits.) This makes the toy safe for most children but will not foil the really determined! Cut off the stopper and the little strip of plastic which joins it to the nozzle, in case this is chewed. Toddlers like to squirt jets of smelly air in their faces and this toy gives good practise in squeezing.

Some children love to concoct 'bad' smells, mixing together perhaps vinegar and a drop of peppermint essence or any other unlikely combination of strong (safe) smells. It also gives them great pleasure to see a grown up sniff such an evil concoction and pull a face over it!

Smells can also be added to favourite soft toys or to fabric collages. The teacher at the deaf-blind unit described on page 81 uses bunches of paper handkerchieves for a section of her feely snake, and sprinkles these with perfume.

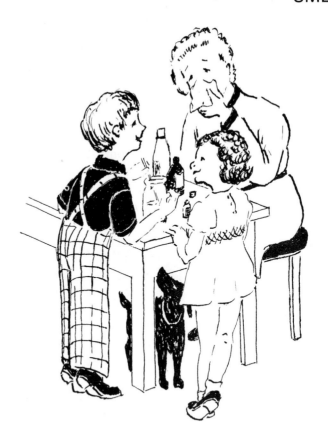

HOME MADE SMELLY TOYS

These can be very quickly created, but are not toys which are made to last because the perfumes will soon fade. Even so they can make a happy diversion on a wet day, or for a sick or bored child. As with all home made toys, they can be devised to be particularly appealing to the individual likes of the child for whom they are made. Some like flowery scents, and a small drop of perfume can provide this. Others prefer very distinctive smells like vinegar and peppermint. Liquid smells can be made more manageable by sprinkling them on a little pad of cotton wool or absorbent paper. Only use a very small amount of any essence partly to avoid waste, but mainly because strong smells—even nice ones—can give a very unpleasant sensation. Some pungent ones, e.g. Eucalyptus oil, if smelt too vigorously could

143

discourage a child from ever sniffing again! Aim at an aroma rather than a smell. An easy way to produce this is to take one or two drops from a bottle by poking the end of a drinking straw just below the level of the liquid. Put your finger firmly over the other end of the straw, lift it out of the bottle, hold it over the pad you want to perfume and release your finger. The liquid will instantly fall where you choose. Children love doing this. Smells can also be diluted by adding them to a damp pad, and this can then be put in a tin with holes in the lid, (or wrapped in a scrap of material) to make it easier to handle.

Smelly Rattles

Make these by putting a few bathsalts in a tin, punching a few holes in the lid (making sure the rough edges are inside) and securely fastening it on again. Plastic pepper pots, well washed, make lovely rattles for small hands and can contain a few coffee beans, or perhaps a little rice to make a noise and a clove to add the smell. This sort of rattle will almost certainly be mouthed and dribbled on, so its life may well be short and busy. If it has added to a baby's experience and enjoyment it will have been worth the little trouble involved in making it.

Smelly Tins for Older Children

Collect a few identical tins or plastic pots with lids. As with the pairs of rattles described on page 69 it is important for the containers to look the same or the child will soon learn to name the contents by the appearance of the container rather than by using his nose. If you want to use the tins on more than one occasion keep the lid as a seal. When the child is identifying the smell, remove the lid, replacing it firmly when the game is over. If the tins are not going to be preserved for another day punch a few holes in the lid and the child can sniff through these.

Smelly Bags

Make these from small balls of cotton wool wrapped up in squares of old rag, and tie them up with string. Liquids can be sprinkled on the cotton wool, and powders like ground cinnamon or crushed up bath salts can be buried in the centre of the ball. The finished bags must *look* as nearly alike as you can make them.

It is often possible for a child to make these smelly

144

bags if he is given some help. This gives him the opportunity of handling the substances and associating them with their smell.

GAMES TO PLAY WITH
SMELLY TINS OR BAGS

Match the Pairs   Make two for each smell and let the child pair them up.

Spot the Stranger   Fill some containers with the same food smell and put something like toothpaste or soap in the 'Stranger' container.

Kim's Game for Smells   Place some different smelly bags on a tray. The child identifies each one. He closes his eyes and one smell is removed. He must then sniff all the bags again and name the missing one.

A harder version of this game can be played by arranging the 'smells' in a circle. The child identifies each. He closes his eyes and the position of the two bags in the circle are exchanged. The child must identify the smells which have been moved.

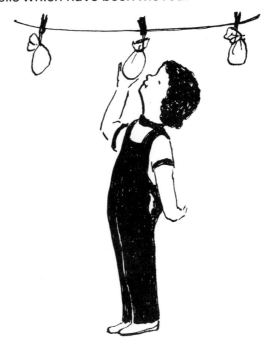

PLAY HELPS

Hang Out the Washing

The child pegs smelly bags at wide intervals along a low hung washing line, pegging the bags about level with his nose. He must then fetch whichever smell he is asked for.

Hunt the Smell

Played like Hunt the Thimble, but a smelly bag is hidden for the child to find.

SMELLY GIFTS FOR A CHILD TO MAKE

Lavender Bags

Children love making these and they are acceptable presents for relatives and friends. Any thin material will do for the bag, but one with small holes in, such as fine net curtain or muslin is nice because the lavender seeds inside can be seen. The simplest lavender bag is made by putting a little pile of lavender in the centre of a square (sides about 6" long) or a circle of material about the size of a tea plate. Tie the lavender up firmly with a length of pretty ribbon. One little girl who spent long hours lying on her tummy, liked to fill a little bag like a tiny pillow case, using a spoon to shovel in the lavender. She would tie this up and fray out the top of the bag to make a decorative fringe.

Pommanders

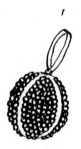

These make splendid smelly Christmas presents but must be started in good time to allow them to dry out. They need to be decorated with plenty of cloves so are not cheap to make. Cloves can be bought at some grocers and chemists. Choose a well shaped orange or lemon. Mark it vertically into four segments with narrow strips of Sellotape. This shows where the ribbon will eventually go and defines the areas to be covered with cloves. Make a little hole in the orange with a fine knitting needle or a cocktail stick and poke in a clove until each segment is completely filled. (Care must be taken not to make the hole too deep or to squeeze the orange or the juice will squirt out.) Roll the pommander in a mixture of ground orris root (from a chemist) and ground cinnamon and wrap it in foil or waxed paper from a cereal packet. Keep it in a warm cupboard for about six weeks while it dries out and shrinks. Finally remove the Sellotape and tie up with pretty ribbon.

Appendices

A: BASIC RECIPES

Bubbles

Make your own bubble mixture from washing up liquid and a little water. Add some glycerine or cooking oil (about a teaspoonful to a cup of bubble mixture) and the bubbles will be stronger and more colourful.

Cheap Paste for Scrap Books etc.

Use about half a cup of flour. Mix this with cold water until it is like thin cream. Bring it slowly to the boil, stirring all the time to prevent lumps. This paste is for immediate use and if left will soon go mouldy. A few drops of oil of cloves or peppermint will keep it fresh for longer, and could add to your child's enjoyment by giving the paste a pleasant smell.

Finger Paint

Use the flour and water paste described above, or use starch or cornflour to make the base for the paint. Four tablespoons of starch will need one pint of water to make a paste of the right consistency. Put the powder in a basin and use a little of the cold water to mix it into a stiff paste with no lumps in it. Boil the rest of the water and add it gradually to the paste, stirring all the time. Boil the mixture until it is clear and thick. Leave it to cool and then divide it among several containers. Add a different powder paint to each.

A Small Inking Pad for Printing

Use a tin with a lid, such as a tobacco tin or one that has contained cough sweets. Cut a small piece of foam rubber to fit in the base of the tin and pour onto this some powder paint mixed fairly stiffly with water and a little glycerine. Remember to replace the tin lid after the printing session and the pad should remain usable for quite a while.

Thick Paint for Covering on Cartons.

Use half a cup of powder paint and one tablespoon of soap flakes. Mix into a thick paste with water. Or

147

instead of soap flakes you can mix up the powder paint with equal parts of washing up liquid and water.

Play Pastry

This is a very good tempered recipe and the quantities of materials used need not be very exact. The following amounts make a very satisfactory mixture. To two cups of flour add about half a cup of salt. This helps to keep the dough fresh for longer. Add about two teaspoons of cooking oil and enough water to make a mixture like real pastry. Roll and squeeze the dough to make sure it is thoroughly mixed together. If it is at all sticky, add a little more flour. To make a change sometimes add powder paint or food colouring to the dough. It can be stored in a fridge in a polythene bag and will easily stay fresh for a week.

B: PLAY FOR THE OLDER HANDICAPPED CHILD

The natural increase in physical size that growing up will inevitably bring often means that a handicapped child can tend to become more and more housebound just because it is now that much more difficult to lift him in and out of cars, help him on buses or trundle his heavy wheelchair up and down steps. Sometimes such confinement cannot be helped but on these occasions the inevitable problems of boredom and loneliness must be overcome. Some parents encourage their child to develop a skill which others like to share, and have found that games or a common interest can be excellent ways of bringing children together and forming friendships. If you were to knock on a certain front door on a Wednesday evening after school, you would find Colin (who has muscular dystrophy) engrossed in a battle of Chess with the retired gentleman who lives next door. In another part of the town, Peter (who has badly injured his foot, and is home between operations,) spends his evenings in the hall of his house playing darts with his friends. Sarah is mentally handicapped but her toy shelf contains several dice games which rely on luck (not speed) for winning and she often enjoys these with her young sister and her friend. Michael has an electric railway and Peter a large

APPENDICES

football game where the teams are made to kick the ball by rotating large knobs. Such toys act as magnets to the other boys in the road, so these two seldom lack for company. Anne cannot walk, but she has learnt to play the guitar and she and her friend sometimes make a tape recording to send to another girl who has left their school.

Many boys and girls may have plenty of interests while they are at school but holidays, weekends and perhaps bouts of illness may make time hang heavily on their hands. They would welcome a hobby, but so far have not found one within their capabilities which really interests them. One of the organisations listed on page 152 might suggest a suitable club, or a book from the following list could provide a possible solution.

C: BOOKS
BOOKS ON THINGS FOR OLDER CHILDREN TO DO

General Interest

Something to Do
Septima Penguin 1966
Suggested games, pastimes and hobbies for every month of the year.
What Shall I do To-day?
What Shall I do With This?
Both by Margaret Hutchings Mills and Boon 1965
Holiday Treasures
Published by Mills and Boon 1971
Describes how to paint pebbles, eggshells, or make paper flowers etc.
Starting Points
Edited by Henry Pluckrose Evans.
These are a series of books on a wide range of subjects eg printing, modelling, puppetry, cooking etc designed for children to use by themselves. Materials needed for each activity are listed, and these are clear instructions and suggestions for more things to do.
Hobbies for Juniors
Peter Arkwright An Arco Handbook
Ideas for active children, but also suggestions for various collections which might interest physically handicapped children.
The Art and Craft Book
Compiled by Henry Pluckrose Evans 1970
Many traditional ideas, and some unusual ones too. eg blowing paint!
Collecting Things
Elizabeth Gundrey Piccolo 1974

Games

101 Best Card Games for Children
Alfred Sheinwood Kaye and Ward 1974
Games for Trains Planes and Wet Days
Gyles Brandreth William Luscombe 1974
How to Amuse Yourself on a Journey
Judy Allen Studio Vista 1974
Illustrated Chess for Children
Harvey Kidder Sidgwick and Jackson 1972
Chess for You
The Easy book for Beginners.
Robert S. Fenton Macdonald 1973

Hobbies

Carpentry is Easy When You Know How
A Golden Hands Junior Book 1974
Coin Collecting A Beginner's Guide
R. F. Johnson Lutterworth Press 1970
Coin Collecting
Joseph Grafton Milne Oxford University Press 1950

Your Book of Coin Collecting
Peter Alan Rayner Faber and Faber 1970
How coinage began, how to start a collection, house it clean it and build it up.
Fishing An illustrated Introduction to the Art of Catching Fish
Nelson Young World 1970
The Art of Angling
Trevor R. Housley Evans 1965
A guide to fresh and salt water fishing.
Flower Pressing
Peter and Susanne Bauzen Little Craft Book Series.
Oak Tree Press 1972
How to do it, and how to use the pressed flowers as decorations.
Folding Paper Puppets
Shari Lewis and Lillian Oppenheimer
Frederick Muller 1971
Paper Cutting
Florence Temko Worlds Work 1974
Origami
Robert Harbin Illustrated Teach Yourself Book.
Brockhampton Press 1973
How to Make and Fly Kites
Eve Barwell and Conrad Bailey Studio Vista 1972
Rag Bag Treasures
Published by Mills and Boon 1971
Toys sewn from odd bits and pieces.
Sewing Things
Elizabeth Gundrey Piccolo 1974
My Learn to Sew Book
Janet Barber Hamlyn
Dolls and How to Make Them
Margaret Hutchings Mills and Boon 1963
Using Fabrics for Fun
Alice White Mills and Boon 1971
Beginner's Guide to Stamp Collecting
Colin Narbeth Lutterworth Press 1966
Stamp Collecting
L. N. and M. Williams Brockhampton Press 1972
Stars and Space
Patrick Moore Black 1969
A clear and simple introduction to astronomy with plenty of illustrations.
Making Things Together
Kathleen Douet and Valerie Jackson Pelham Books 1973
A particularly valuable book of ideas for things to make and to play with. The activities need varying amounts of skill, so parents and more able children can tackle the difficult parts while the simple jobs can be managed by the less experienced!

BOOKS ON TOYS AND PLAY

Play With a Purpose for the Under Sevens
E.M. Matterson   Penguin
Written primarily for playgroup leaders this book is full of practical suggestions for constructive play.

Playing, Learning and Living
Vera Roberts   A.C. Black   1971
Shows how children usually go through various stages of play.

Play Activities for the Retarded Child
Carlson and Ginglend   Abingdon Press   1961
Full of sensible and enjoyable activities often graded in difficulty so that one elementary skill learnt can be used in the next stage.

Discovering With Young Children
Ash, Win and Hutchinson   Elek   1971
As the title suggests, this book has a slightly scientific slant and gives play ways of helping children to find out about weight, texture, wind, etc. Natural materials are used a great deal and there are some clearly illustrated reminders of how to make simple traditional toys like paper windmills and hats.

What to do When There's Nothing to do
Members of the Boston Children's Medical Centre   Hutchinson   1972
This book is arranged by age group and gives helpful, easily carried out suggestions on how to combat boredom from babyhood onwards.

Mother's Help
Edited by Susan Dickinson   Collins   1972
Chapters on different subjects such as gardening, story telling, music, dressing up, cooking etc. are each written by a different expert.

175 Ideas to Keep Children Happy
A Golden Hands Special

Pre School Play
Kenneth Jameson and Pat Kidd   Studio Vista   1974

CHILD DEVELOPMENT

Baby Learning Through Baby Play
Child Learning Through Child Play
Both by Dr. Ina Gordon
Sidgwick and Jackson   1973
The Developmental Progress of Infants and Young Children
Dr. Mary D. Sheridan   H.M.S.O.   1968

Your Child's First Five Years
Martin Bax and Judy Bernal   Heinemann Health Books   1974

Book of Child Care
Hugh Jolly   Allen and Unwin   1975

BOOKS PARTICULARLY HELPFUL TO PARENTS OF HANDICAPPED CHILDREN

Handicapped Children
John D. Kershaw   William Heinemann Medical Books Ltd.   1973
This book gives information on all handicaps and what they can mean in terms of daily living. Assessment, schooling and the best possibilities of employment are all discussed.

The Young Handicapped Child
A. H. Bowley   Livingstone

Caring for Your Disabled Child
B. Spock and M. O. Lerrigo   Macmillan   1965
This is an American book, but it contains plenty of helpful information for parents of any nationality. Eg. Part V is headed 'Enjoying Life' and deals with play, clubs and activities, and Part VII gives practical advice on caring for artificial limbs, aids, braces etc.

Early Years
Morigue Cornwell   Disabled Living Foundation, 346 Kensington High Street, London, W14 8NS

Aids for the Severely Handicapped
Ed. Keith Copeland   Sector Publishing   1974
Twenty nine contributors describe devices they have made which have helped people with very little movement to be more independent and to communicate more easily.

Clothing for the Handicapped Child
Available from the Disabled Living Foundation, 346 Kensington High Street, London W14 8NS

Life and Leisure for the Physically Handicapped
Ruth Elliott   Elek   1971
Concerned mainly with the needs of adults, but also useful for teenagers.

Handbook for Parents with a Handicapped Child
Judith Stone and Felicity Taylor   CASE Publications
17 Jackson's Lane, Billericay, Essex.
A list of addresses of organizations covering the needs of all handicaps.

Spotlight on Services for the Young Handicapped Child
Jesse Parfitt   National Children's Bureau   1972
Adam House, 1 Fitzroy Square, London, W1P 5AH

Handling the Young Cerebral Palsied Child at Home
Nancie R. Finnie   Heinemann   1974

The Challenge of Spina Bifida
Alan Field   Heinemann   1970
Spina Bifida explained for parents. Advice on overcoming all the problems.

Spina Bifida The Treatment and Care of Spina Bifida Children.
Nancy Allum   Allen and Unwin   1975

APPENDICES

Helping the Trainable Mentally Retarded Child Develop Speech and Language
G. Thomas Gordon Ryan and Shilo
A guide for parents.
Teaching the Retarded Child to Talk
Julia S. Molloy University of London Press 1965
Language Stimulus with Retarded Children
Mary la Frenais National Society for Mentally Handicapped children, Pembridge Hall, 17, Pembridge Square, London, W2 4EP.
On Helping the Dyslexic Child
T. R. Miles Methuen 1970

Learning to Talk
Margaret Greene Heinemann
Language Through Play
Patricia Denner Arno Press
The Hearing Impaired Child Under Five
Sir Alexander Ewing and Lady Ethel c. Ewing Manchester University Press 1971
A guide for parents and teachers.
Learning to Hear A Special Revision for Parents
E. Whetnall and D. B. Fry Heinemann
Deaf Children at Home and School
D. M. C. Dale University of London Press

PLAY FOR SICK CHILDREN

Play in Hospital
Susan Harvey and Ann Hales Tooke Faber 1972
Play and the Sick Child
Eva Noble Faber 1967
Toys and Ideas for Children When Ill
A leaflet published by James Galt and Co. Ltd., Brookfield Road, Cheadle, Cheshire.

Games to Play for the Sick Child
G. and C. Kay Corgi Mini Books Transworld 1972
Written by a doctor and a nurse, this little book is full of practical hints and ideas for all ages and all stages of illness from 'very poorly' to 'nearly well'.
Stay in Bed Book
Inger Bassingthwaite Studio Vista 1974

BOOKS ABOUT HANDICAPPED PEOPLE

The Child Who Never Grew
Pearl S. Buck Methuen
About a mentally retarded child.
Born That Way
Earl Carlson Evesham James
About a spastic who qualifies as a doctor.
The Small Outsider
Joan Martin Hundley Angus and Robertson 1971
About Autism
I Can't See What You're Saying
Elizabeth Browning Elek
About a deaf, aphasic child.
Blind Man's Buff
H. Minton Garland
The experiences of a middle aged man who suddenly becomes blind.
The Story of My Life
Hellen Keller Hodder
The autobiography of a remarkable deaf blind lady.
Teacher
Anne Sullivan Macey Gollancz
Written by Helen Keller's teacher
Child of Gentle Courage
Sarah Shears Elek 1974
The story of a country child who is run over and suffers brain damage. Her progress through childhood, her fight for independence and her marriage.
The Small Outsider
Joan Martin Hundley Angus and Robertson 1971
The story of an autistic child.

D: ADDRESSES OF ORGANIZATIONS CONCERNED WITH PLAY AND LEISURE TIME ACTIVITIES

The Toy Libraries Association, Sunley House, Gunthorpe Street, London, E1 7RW.
Write for latest list of T.L.A. booklets on play for handicapped children with many differing needs.
The Pre-School Playgroups Association, Alfred House, Aveline Street, London, S.E.11
345 Ltd. 92a, Old Street London, ECIV9AY
(For a twelve month course of nursery education to be used at home. Each month a fresh batch of material arrives.)
John Tracey Clinic, 806 West Adam Boulevard, Los Angeles, California 90007, U.S.A.
(For a correspondance course for parents of pre-school deaf children.)
Riding for the Disabled Secretary and Treasurer, Miss S.L. Thompson, Brockhurst Lodge, 31 Shortheath Road, Farnham, Surrey.
The National Association of Swimming Clubs for the Handicapped, 93 The Downs, Harlow, Essex.
Extension Guiding, The Deputy Training Secretary, 17-19, Buckingham Palace Road, London, S.W.1.
Extension Scouting, The Activities Secretary, The Scout Association, Gillwell Park, Chingford, London, E47QW
National Playing Fields Association 57b, Catherine Place, London, S.W.1.

(Keeps a national register of adventure playgrounds for the handicapped.
Breakthrough, 3, Cocksett Avenue, Orpington, Kent.
(Arranges family holidays for deaf and multi-handicapped deaf children, and also organises outings etc.)
Disabled Living Foundation, 346, Kensington High Street, London, W14 8NS.
(For information on aids of every kind, from wheel chairs and stair hoists to how to tie up your shoes without using a bow!)
London for the Disabled by Freda Bruce Lockhart   Ward Lock   1971
(Gives information on car parking, toilets, restaurants, easy access to buildings etc. Particularly useful to parents whose children are in wheelchairs.)

E: TOY MANUFACTURERS AND SUPPLIERS WHO WILL SEND CATALOGUES AND DEAL THROUGH MAIL ORDERS

Abbatt Toys 74, Wigmore Street, London, W.1.
(Also through E.S.A.)
John Adams Toys Ltd Mail Order Department, Crazies Hill, Wargrave, Berks.
(Wooden toys of all sizes, games and puzzles—some specially suitable for children with handicaps. Eg. Klik, a game like Spillikins where little sticks must be extricated from a pile without disturbing it. Klik has tiny magnets incorporated in the pieces and is specially good for older children needing a "low effort" toy.)
Albion Nursery Goods Ltd. 3, Clem Atlee Parade, London, SW6 7RJ.
(Particularly recommended for a large stock of mobiles.)
Anything Left Handed Ltd. 65, Beek Street, London, W.1.
E. J. Arnold and Son Ltd. Butterley Street, Leeds, LS10 1AX.
(Educational Suppliers)
Bagatelle (Toys) Ltd. 7, Gun Street, Reading, Berks.
(For toys, games and things to do for all ages. Specially for giant playing cards which are easier for some children to see and for others to hold.)
Community Playthings, Carvell, Robertsbridge, Sussex, TN32 5DR.
(For very strong wooden toys, all guaranteed for one year.)
E.S.A. (Educational Supply Association) Pinnacles, P.O. Box 22, Harlow, Essex, CM19 5AY
(This firm produces two catalogues particularly useful to parents of handicapped children;
    (a) Play Specials
    (b) Extra Specials (for larger and older children.)
They also supply Carl Orff percussion instruments etc.)
Escor Toys Grovely Road, Christchurch, Hants BH23 3RQ
Four to Eight, Medway House, St. Mary's Mills, Evelyn Drive, Leicester, LE3 2BT.
Gallery Five Ltd, 14, Ogle Street London, WIP 7LG.
(For children's posters and friezes.)
James Galt and Co. P.O. Box 2, Cheadle, Cheshire.

(Toys and play materials for all ages.)
Gazelle Toys Ltd, Snedshill Trading Estate, Oakengates, Telford, Shropshire.
(For specially light aluminium toys, eg. stilts weighing 3 lb, and a baby walker weighing 2½lb.)
Good-Wood Toys (Lavant) Ltd., Chichester, Sussex.
(For strong wooden toys from bricks to Wendy houses. Specially for Plan a Village—a game controlled by magnets specially suitable for children with limited movement or for bed play.)
Hamleys of Regent Street, 200-202, Regent Street, London, WIR 5DF.
(A huge toy shop which can supply a wide range of toys.)
Happy Things, 4 Babbington Village, Eastwood, Nottinghamshire.
(For inexpensive children's posters and white plastic hangers to suspend them by.)
Thomas Hope Ltd., St. Philip's Drive, Royton Oldham, Lancashire.
(Educational Suppliers. For toys, games, art equipment etc.)
Huntercraft P.O.Box 1, Stalbridge, Dorset.
(A small firm particularly interested in making toys for handicapped children.)
Learning Development Aids, Park Works, Norwich Road, Wisbech, Cambs, PE13 2AX.
(Materials for children with learning difficulties.)
David Lethbridge, The Bakehouse, Northchapel, Petworth, Sussex.
(For wooden toys—some large, some recommended as "Stocking fillers".)
London Music Shop, 218, Great Portland Street, London, WIN 6JH
(For instruments, tutors, music, song books etc.)
Philip and Tacey Ltd., Northway, Andover, Hants.
(Educational Suppliers. Specially good for tough books on a spiral spine. Eg. Three of a Kind Strip Books. Each page has been cut into three strips and these can be arranged to make a set or three related pictures.)
Postal Playthings, P.O.Box 23, 180, Drury Lane, London, W.C.2.

APPENDICES

(For cheaper novelty toys. Particularly for a set of eight large tough space age stencils, ideal for small boys.)

R.N.I.B. (Royal National Institute for the Bline) 224-6-8, Great Portland Street, London, W.1.

(For catalogue of apparatus and games specially for the blind.)

Toy and Furniture Workshop, Church Hill, Totland Bay, Isle of Wight.

345 Kiddicraft,

Books records and games for pre-school children. Available from large toy shops, W.H.Smiths, department stores etc.

Tridias, 8 Saville Row, Bath.

Toys by post.

Woodpecker Toys Ltd., Burvill Street, Lynton, North Deven

(Both for strong wooden toys.)

F: ADDRESSES OF ORGANIZATIONS CONCERNED WITH HANDICAPPED CHILDREN

Association for all Speech Impaired Children
Hon. Sec. Mrs J. Rankin, 9 Desenfans Road, Dulwich Village, London, SE21 7DN

Association for Spina Bifida and Hydrocephalus
Devonshire Street House, 30 Devonshire Street, London, W1N 2EB

The British Deaf Association or Teenagers and Young Adults
38 Victoria Place, Carlisle CA1 1EX

British Diabetic Association
3-6 Alfred Place, London, WC1E 7EE

British Dyslexia Association
18, The Circus, Bath, BA1 2ET

British Epilepsy Association
3-6 Alfred Place, London, WC1E 7EE

Brittle Bone Society
Secretary and Treasurer Mrs M. Grant, 63 Byron Crescent, Dundee, Scotland

Children's Chest Circle,
Tavistock House North, Tavistock Square, London WC1

Downs Babies Association
Quinborne Community Centre, Ridgacre Road, Quinton, Birmingham, B32 2TW

Invalid Children's Aid Association
126 Buskingham Palace Road, London, SW1W 9SB

National Association for Deaf/Blind and Rubella Children
61 Senneleys Park Road, Northfield, Birmingham, B31 1AE

National Association for the Welfare of Children in Hospital
7 Exton Street, London, SE1 8VE

National Deaf Children's Society
31 Gloucester Place, London, W1

National Society for Autistic Children
1a Golders Green Road, London, NW11

National Society for Mentally Handicapped Children
Pembridge Hall, 17 Pembridge Square, London W2 4EP

Muscular Dystrophy Group of Great Britain
26 Borough High Street, London, SE1

Royal National Institute for the Blind
224 Great Portland Street, London, W1

Royal National Institute for the Deaf
105 Gower Street, London, WC1E 6AH

Spastics Society
12 Park Crescent, London, W1N 4EQ

INDEX